Caring for Patients at
the End of Life

Caring for Patients at the End of Life

Facing an Uncertain Future Together

TIMOTHY E. QUILL, M.D.

Professor of Medicine, Psychiatry, and Medical Humanities
University of Rochester School of Medicine and Dentistry
Program for Biopsychosocial Studies
Rochester, New York

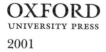

OXFORD
UNIVERSITY PRESS

2001

OXFORD
UNIVERSITY PRESS

Oxford   New York
Athens   Auckland   Bangkok   Bogotá   Buenos Aires   Calcutta
Cape Town   Chennai   Dar es Salaam   Delhi   Florence   Hong Kong   Istanbul
Karachi   Kuala Lumpur   Madrid   Melbourne   Mexico City   Mumbai
Nairobi   Paris   São Paulo   Shanghai   Singapore   Taipei   Tokyo   Toronto   Warsaw

and associated companies in
Berlin   Ibadan

Published by Oxford University Press, Inc.
198 Madison Avenue, New York, New York 10016

Oxford is a registered trademark of Oxford University Press

Library of Congress Cataloging-in-Publication Data
Quill, Timothy E.
      Caring for patients at the end of life: facing an uncertain future together /
Timothy E. Quill.
      p.; cm.   Includes bibliographical references and index.
      ISBN 0-19-513940-2 (paper)
      1. Terminal care.   2. Palliative treatment.   3. Physician and patient.
   I. Title
      [DNLM: 1. Terminal Care—methods.
   2. Attitude to Death.   3. Palliative Care—methods.
   WB 310 Q6c 2001]   R726.8 .Q548 2001   362.1'75—dc21   00-062437

The science of medicine is a rapidly changing field. As new research and clinical experience
broaden our knowledge, changes in treatment and drug therapy do occur. The author and the
publisher of this work have checked with sources believed to be reliable in their efforts to
provide information that is accurate and complete, and in accordance with the standards
accepted at the time or publication. However, in light of the possibility of human error or
changes in the practice of medicine, neither the author, nor the publisher, nor any other party
who has been involved in the preparation or publication of this work warrants that the information contained herein is in every respect accurate or complete. Readers are encouraged to
confirm the information contained herein with other reliable sources, and are strongly advised
to check the product information sheet provided by the pharmceutical company for each drug
they plan to administer.

9 8 7 6 5 4 3 2 1

Printed in the United States of America
on acid-free paper

In Memory of My Brother
Don Quill
1/23/57–4/14/00

And

In Honor of His Son
David John
8/19/99

Foreword

Nearly a decade ago, Dr. Timothy E. Quill submitted a short paper to the *New England Journal of Medicine*, of which I was then Executive Editor. The paper, titled "Death and Dignity: A Case of Individualized Decision-Making," told the story of Diane, a woman who had been Dr. Quill's patient for 8 years and now faced a protracted death from leukemia. She asked Quill for the means to take her own life if she found the dying process unbearable. She needed the possibility of escape. Quill gave her a prescription for a large dose of barbiturates. Four months later, faced with a sudden downhill course after a period of peace and contentment, Diane took the pills Quill had prescribed and ended her life.

I was impressed by the simple, affecting way in which Quill told the story (reprinted here as Chapter 3) and by his overriding commitment to help Diane meet death on her own terms, despite the obvious torment that caused him. And I was just as impressed by his courage. When I finished reading the paper, I knew I wanted to publish it, yet I was concerned for Quill. Physician-assisted suicide was illegal in New York, and it seemed to me that his paper might be considered a public confession of a crime. I telephoned him and suggested he take a few days to think about the possible consequences to him of publishing Diane's story. He seemed a little surprised, but agreed. Three days later, he told me very calmly that he felt the story of Diane raised issues that needed to be discussed openly, and he was willing to take whatever personal risks that entailed. (Quill was in fact brought before a grand jury, which had the wisdom not to indict him.)

That was the beginning of Quill's remarkable career as a thoughtful and elo-quent spokesman for dying patients and for the doctors who care for them. He has written several books on the subject, and was a plaintiff in *Quill v. Vacco*, one of two important cases to reach the U. S. Supreme Court in 1997 arguing for the right of physician-assisted suicide. Despite the fact that the Court found no such right, the decision focused attention on the inadequacies of care at the end of life and the necessity to address them.

Quill does that here, in a book that few will be able to put down once they start it. What happens when we find that a deadly disease cannot be cured, when the best that can be hoped for is a reasonably comfortable and peaceful death? Suppose even that is elusive, that with the best palliative care possible, death is still an unremitting and prolonged agony? Using as illustrations the compelling stories of patients he or his colleagues have cared for, Quill answers these and other questions in this comprehensive exploration of care at the end of life.

In the first part of the book, Quill deals with underlying values and assump-tions. In particular, he stresses the need for doctors to form a partnership with dying patients to find the best death based on each particular patient's values. Most important, he discusses the necessity of doctors staying the course, no matter how difficult, so that dying patients are never abandoned.

In the second (and best, in my view) part, Quill brilliantly illustrates the kinds of conversations that should take place between doctors and dying patients. By emphasizing the importance of listening and learning from the patient, he shows how to deliver bad news in the most honest, compassionate, and con-structive way. He also shows how to broach the subject of shifting the empha-sis from curative to palliative care, and how to evaluate and respond to requests for help in dying. Obviously, such conversations take time and concentrated attention, an effort not well rewarded in this day of managed care and high technology medicine. Yet, Quill shows just how important it is.

In the third part, Quill discusses the challenging clinical and ethical issues that arise in terminal illness as suffering increases and death becomes immi-nent. He makes it clear that while excellent palliative care in a hospice setting can relieve most symptoms, it cannot relieve all of them, particularly the debil-itation and dependency many patients find so hard to endure. He also points out that the philosophy of hospice, with its emphasis on dying as an opportu-nity for personal growth, is not for everyone. Suppose, despite the best pallia-tive care, suffering is largely unrelieved and the patient asks to die faster? What then?

Quill discusses how to evaluate such a request and presents in an easy-to-understand, yet comprehensive way the options for relieving intractable suffering and bringing about a faster death. These include increasing the doses of opioids, even at the risk of hastening death; withholding life-sustaining treatment, such as antibiotics; sedating the patient to unconsciousness, then withholding intravenous feeding until death; suggesting that the patient voluntarily stop eating and drinking until death; physician-assisted suicide; and voluntary active euthanasia. Quill discusses each method, its legal and ethical status, and its philosophical underpinnings. In doing so, he readily challenges conventional wisdom about such matters as whether the 13th century theological doctrine of double effect is really necessary to justify administering life-threatening doses of opioids, whether terminal sedation is really morally distinct from euthanasia, and whether ceasing to eat and drink causes undue suffering in an already desperate patient. The reader is left with the impression that some of the widely accepted ethical analyses are not only tortuous, but simply ways of circumventing the legal prohibitions against physician-assisted suicide and euthanasia.

Quill ends the book with a poignant chapter about the death of his brother, just at the time Quill was finishing the book. Although Don Quill did not die a lingering death (he died two days after a bicycle accident), Quill and the rest of his family had to deal with many of the same painful issues as families of terminally ill patients. Quill makes us feel with full force how he experienced those issues.

This book should be read not only by ordinary Americans, but also by doctors and nurses who care for dying patients. All of us face the possibility of a lingering death, and most of us have family members or friends who have died such a death. If we can't all have Tim Quill as a doctor, the next best thing would be to have a doctor who has read his book.

Marcia Angell, M.D.
Former Editor-in-Chief, *New England Journal of Medicine*
Senior Lecturer in Social Medicine, Harvard Medical School

Acknowledgments

This book is a work of collaboration—with my patients, their families, my colleagues, and my family. The clinical narratives that form the heart of this book are based on real patients whose lives and deaths I have had the privilege to share. I continue to marvel at the meaning and importance of end-of-life clinical work, and how central it is to medicine's mission. I thank these patients and their families for allowing me to disclose some aspects their end-of-life experiences in the hopes of teaching others about what is possible during this remarkable time of life, especially if we work together with honesty, caring, compassion, and courage.

Several chapters are based on articles that were co-authored by colleagues who have been on the forefront of articulating new approaches to end-of-life care—Chris Cassel, Bernie Lo, James Tulsky, Jason Karlawish, Diane Meier, Dan Brock, and Rebecca Dresser. Although I take full responsibility for all alterations and additions to these articles, I am grateful to them for generously allowing me to build on many of the ideas that we collaboratively developed in these original manuscripts.

Marcia Angell, the author of the book's foreword, was the editor of the *New England Journal of Medicine* when I submitted my original narrative about Diane's life and death. I thank her for having the foresight to accept the manuscript for publication, and for her subsequent collaboration and support over

xii   **Acknowledgments**

the years. The painting reproduced on the book cover is by Marcia Smith, a wonderful artist and friend who also is living with advanced illness.

The development, editing, and production also required collaboration. My wife, Penny, was involved in all phases of the book, from conceptualization to early editing to fine-tuning. Maria Milella, my administrative assistant and trusted colleague, has worked tirelessly helping with the details of research, editing, and production. Finally, Lauren Enck and her colleagues at Oxford University Press have been professional and generous with their guidance and support, and a pleasure to work with—a relatively rare combination. The final manuscript is truly the collective product of many hands, hearts, and minds.

Finally, with my brother's untimely death, 2000 was the hardest of years for our family. Yet, despite our anguish and grief, we have pulled together as a family, and in that sense joined with the other families in the book in trying to make sense of our loss. Telling our story in the Epilogue of this book has helped me to come to terms with Don's death. I want to finally thank my parents Millie and Joe, Don's wife Toni, our brother Steve, my wife Penny, and my children Carrie and Megan for their love and support, and for helping to shape our story. At times like this, you relearn the importance of family, friends, and colleagues you can count on. I am blessed on all accounts.

T.E.Q.
Rochester, N.Y.

Contents

Part 3. Difficult Clinical and Ethical Issues

Caring for Patients at
the End of Life

Introduction

Challenges and Potential of
End-of-Life Care

Imagine the unimaginable. You have just survived a sudden cardiac death. You were quickly resuscitated, and your mind and heart have recovered unscathed. Your sense of who you are as a person, however, will never be the same. Some difficult questions inevitably emerge:

- *Why did this happen to me at this particular time?*
- *What can I do to prevent it from occurring again?*
- *If it happens again, will I survive intact?*
- *What if my body survives but my brain does not?*
- *What will happen to my family if I die, or become severely impaired?*
- *What happens to me after I die?*

These questions and others were being frantically considered by Mrs. W. when I first met her about 15 years ago at the age of 68. Mrs. W. had been widowed for 20 years. Her sense of self had evolved considerably since her husband's death, as she learned to take charge of all household and personal affairs. Up until her cardiac arrest, she had been receiving regular medical contact for illnesses such as irritable colon syndrome, diverticulitis, hypertension, and back pain, but never before had she faced a life-threatening illness.

1

Mrs. W. was the sole caretaker of her 25 year-old daughter, Joan. Joan was moderately developmentally disabled, and required daily supervision. With Mrs. W.'s help, Joan was able to manage most of her basic daily activities. Joan also worked several hours per day in a sheltered workshop. She and her mother had a symbiotic relationship, each watching over the other with more skill and energy than they devoted to themselves. Mrs. W.'s main fear after her cardiac arrest was what would become of Joan if she died. Mrs. W. had several other children, but they led successful, active lives with little room for this additional responsibility. They were very willing to help with their sister in the short run, but none of them could commit to her ongoing daily supervision.

Mrs. W. received careful medical evaluation. Her angiogram showed minimal disease in her coronary arteries; her problems appeared to be more electrical than circulatory. She was started on medication that stabilized the rhythm of her heart. At this point, Mrs. W. had an excellent quality of life, and she was willing to do anything possible to preserve and extend it. She was, however, at risk for having another cardiac arrest at any moment, and perhaps not surviving intact. I therefore initiated a discussion on several levels with her and her family.

For example, were there circumstances where she would not want to receive aggressive care, perhaps where she would not find life worth living? Mrs. W. talked about both her intellectual and physical independence—if her quality of life and independence could not be preserved or recovered, she would want all life-prolonging treatment to be stopped. She also spoke about her desire not to linger if and when she was dying. Her husband died a prolonged and difficult death, and the experience was difficult for the entire family. If she had to die, she would prefer to do so painlessly and quickly. Finally, Mrs. W. talked about how she would like us to proceed with the care of her daughter if she were to die or become incapacitated. One of her sons agreed that under such circumstances, he would temporarily take Joan into his home, and then later help find an acceptable group home for her. Her son would continue to oversee Joan's care and well-being, and have her become a bigger part of his family.

Mrs. W. completed a living will articulating her values and wishes in this regard, and her son in town was formally designated as her health care proxy. I acknowledged her sense of unnerving uncertainty in not knowing how her future illness would unfold, and I promised to always keep her values and wishes at center stage. Although these discussions gave increased reality to the possibility of death, Mrs. W. generally found them reassuring. She was relieved to have a clear plan articulated for her family and for me, as her physician, if she became unable to speak for herself in the future.

Although Mrs. W. fully recovered from her cardiac arrest, her self-confidence was somewhat undermined. She and Joan had always loved to travel, particularly to visit members of their large extended family, who lived all over the country. Because of her uncertain medical future, Mrs. W. now felt she should stay close to home in case something happened. Once her medication had been stabilized, my advice to her was to travel freely. If her time was limited, what better way to die than by doing something that she truly treasured? If she had a cardiac arrest away from home, the odds of her surviving would be the same as they would be if she had one in town. Furthermore, living life in continuous fear and anticipation of the next adverse event would not be living.

Mrs. W. took my advice and gradually resumed her active travel schedule. Fortunately, she had no further cardiac events or serious illnesses for the next 10 years, during which time she attended innumerable family events. Unfortunately, when she did have a second cardiac arrest, she was at a family reunion out of state. Once again she was quickly and successfully resuscitated. She was stabilized at a local hospital, and survived with full physical and mental integrity. When she returned home this time, we changed her rhythm-stabilizing medication and tested how well it worked by electrically provoking her heart under controlled circumstances. She also had a permanent cardiac defibrillator implanted in her chest, so she could immediately and automatically be resuscitated should she suffer another cardiac arrest in the future.

It took several months for her to recover, but eventually Mrs. W. was again traveling to family events (albeit at a little slower pace than in the past). She had several more years of high-quality, very independent life before she began to deteriorate. At age 82—15 years after her initial cardiac arrest—Mrs. W. began to fail. It was subtle at first—she exhibited some decreased appetite, a slow decline in weight, vague abdominal pain, and increased weakness. I initially thought she might have a gastrointestinal or pancreatic malignancy, but an extensive medical evaluation did not unearth any cause other than poor circulation to her bowels, which was not amenable to treatment. She eventually lost 50 pounds, and started having frequent falls. Several hospitalizations and medication adjustments did not reverse or stabilize her progressive decline.

Since Mrs. W.'s quality of life was rapidly fading, we discussed placing more emphasis on relief of suffering and less on aggressive testing and treatment. Because she had no clearly defined terminal illness, she did not qualify for a hospice program. Furthermore, she did not want to preclude any treatment that might prolong her life without substantially adding to her suffering. With my guidance, however, she did decide that extremely invasive treatments such as mechanical ventilation, dialysis, or cardiopulmonary resuscitation would be more than she wanted to endure given her current level of debility. Mrs. W. understood that she would be unlikely to return to her current level of function and independence should these treatments be needed. We therefore completed a do-not-resuscitate (DNR) document, but agreed to consider the potential risks and benefits of any other future treatments on a case-by-case basis.

Although Mrs. W. did not fit the admission criteria for a Medicare-sponsored hospice program, we provided her with many of the elements of hospice care. This approach, called "palliative care," is defined as the providing of total care for patients whose disease is not responsive to curative treatment, and includes pain and symptom management as well as psychological, social, spiritual, and existential support for the patient and family.[1] There was no reason to exclude her from this approach simply because she did not have a clearly defined terminal illness, or because she chose to continue some disease-directed medical interventions.

Mrs. W.'s chronic abdominal pain lessened with around-the-clock opioids, and her nausea was suppressed by medication that blocked the secretion of gastric acid. Since it would not be surprising for her to die in the next six months (though it was by no means certain), we talked with Mrs. W. and her family about any parts of her life that would be incomplete if she were to die sooner rather than later. With her son, she reaffirmed the plan that had been set up for Joan, and they began to explore group homes and supports available in the community. I also inquired about unaddressed spiritual or religious issues, which led her to contact her pastor, who began visiting her regularly at home. If we were premature in exploring these issues, nothing would be lost. If we avoided them and she died earlier than anticipated, an important opportunity might have been lost.

There was a lot of uncertainty about how to prepare Joan for her mother's eventual death. I decided to let Joan guide the conversation, and began a cautious exploration about her understanding of her mother's illness. Not surprisingly, Joan knew that her mother was very sick, and was already anticipating that she might die. She was trying to protect her mother by not talking about it, just as her mother was trying to spare her from unnecessary grief. We offered to help them talk together, but neither wanted to, preferring to "protect" and take care of each other in the ways that had worked so well for 35 years. We left the door open for direct contact around these issues, but continued to respect their wishes.

Mrs. W. was virtually wheelchair bound at this point. There was one final family reunion that she wanted to attend, and we made arrangements for her to travel and participate as much as she could. Although she was extremely frail and vulnerable, she pulled herself together for the trip and had a wonderful time. In addition to being a celebration of a grandchild's graduation, the party was a tear-filled yet joyous good-bye for Mrs. W. She returned exhausted, but proud of having made her "final trip." She knew that death was nearby, but hoped to hang on a little longer, as much for Joan as for herself.

Over the next several weeks, Mrs. W. became progressively weaker, and was eventually admitted to the hospital after developing a high fever, shaking chills, and symptoms of a kidney infection. At a family meeting with Mrs. W. present, I recommended a trial of antibiotic treatment in the hope that the infection had contributed to her recent deterioration. The option of allowing the infection to be "the old woman's friend" was also discussed, but Mrs. W. was not prepared to die if she had a condition that might easily be reversed. If her condition did not rapidly improve, she would accept death, and we would devote our energies exclusively to keeping her comfortable. Because death was likely near, family members were called in from out of town.

As expected, Mrs. W. did not improve. Within 36 hours, her blood pressure dropped, her kidney function began deteriorating, and she lost the capacity to speak for herself. Her son and I assembled a meeting of her family, and I recommended an approach devoted exclusively to her comfort. Mrs. W. had made her wishes clear in this regard, and our job now was to carry them out. Having participated in many earlier discussions, Mrs. W.'s family was supportive of the transition. We stopped her antibiotics and discontinued intravenous fluids, which no longer were serving the goal of her comfort. Her around-the-clock pain medications were increased in response to what appeared to be grimaces of pain. Each person was encouraged to say his or her last good-bye. Joan was able to witness her mother lying in a quiet room freed from medical encumbrances and invasions, in what appeared to be a deep sleep. Last rites were given, and everyone was prepared. Everything possible had been done, and Mrs. W. was dying peacefully and quickly, as she had hoped.

Yet there was a loose end that had the capacity to unravel this scene. Mrs. W. had had an electronic defibrillator inserted several years previously. When her heart stopped, this device would repeatedly deliver a large electric shock in an effort to "restart" it. If she were to die quietly and naturally, the defibrillator would need to be electronically deactivated. Mrs. W.'s cardiologist initially was not comfortable "assisting her to die." Following a discussion about what might happen if the device was left activated, the cardiologist reluctantly consented to deprogram the defibrillator. Witnessing Mrs. W.'s deteriorated condition and the peaceful vigil at her bedside, the cardiologist's uncertainty about "letting her die" dissipated.

Mrs. W. died peacefully six hours later. Her desire to live as long as possible, fully engaged with family and friends, had been achieved. The events surrounding her death had remained largely within her control, and she was able to die relatively quickly and peacefully. Her last year had been challenging as she tried to adjust to increasing physical discomfort and dependence, yet she would not have foreshortened it even for one moment. Caring for Joan kept her going during difficult periods. As long as she could do that, Mrs. W. had a reason to continue living. Toward the end, Joan was caring for Mrs. W. as much as Mrs. W. was caring for her. They wanted it no other way.

Joan went to live with her brother for several months after Mrs. W.'s death. She grieved for her mother, but eventually discovered a new life in a group home located near her brother's house. Joan has adjusted to her new surroundings, but regularly speaks about her mother, who she reports is often in her dreams. Joan has no questions or concerns about her mother's death, but simply misses her presence and support. Her reaction in this regard is almost exactly the same as her brothers'. Mrs. W. lived a long and full life, and was able to die with few regrets and almost no unfinished business.

Mrs. W.'s clinical course had many elements that characterize life and death in the modern medical era. She lived for more than 15 years following a major cardiac arrest. Most of that time was associated with an excellent quality of life. She benefited from advanced medical technology, such as new antiarrhymic medications and an implantable defibrillator. She ignored her illness for the vast majority of the time, except when it asserted itself in dramatic fashion with her episodic cardiac arrests.

During the last year of her life, Mrs. W.'s condition changed. She developed a lack of circulation to her bowel that was not reversible and severely interfered with her quality of life. She was at risk of dying at any time, but could also have lived for several years, so her condition did not fall within the usual definition of a terminal illness. Furthermore, she wanted to continue any medical measures that might prolong her life without substantially adding to her suffering. To qualify for the hospice Medicare benefit, a patient must be highly likely to die within six months and be willing to forgo potentially expensive, curative treatments in favor of treatment devoted to symptom relief and comfort.[2,3] Mrs. W. did not meet either of these requirements.

Yet as she became progressively sicker over the last year of her life, Mrs. W. received palliative care, benefiting from hospice-like care without the formal program. The heath care team could not improve the circulation to her bowels, but we did manage to lessen associated pain and nausea with a sophisticated medical regimen. With her other children, we made tentative plans for her developmentally disabled daughter's future. We facilitated home visits from her pastor, who had been unaware of her recent illness. Eventually we set limits on the degree of invasiveness of her care, including her completion of a do-not-resuscitate document. Finally, because Mrs. W. feared a lingering death where she would be out of control of her mental faculties, she completed a living will, named her son as health care proxy, and made sure that he and the rest of the family understood her wishes.

Like most patients, Mrs. W. wanted to live as long as life continued to be meaningful. Toward the end, she was willing to tolerate considerable suffering in the interest of her survival. Yet she wanted reassurance that she would be the one to decide when enough was enough. When her time came to die, she wanted to do so quickly and painlessly. She did not worry about the details of how this might happen—she simply counted on receiving our help if it were needed to help her die peacefully. This reassurance that we would help her escape when and if her suffering became too great helped sustain her in her last year of life. Her clinical course over the last several days of her life included multiple family meetings, activation of her living will and health care proxy documents when she could no longer speak for herself, aggressive symptom management, the withdrawal of antibiotics and fluids, discontinuation of an implantable defibrillator, and finally, a decision not to perform cardiopulmonary resuscitation when she died. In part as a result of this active decision making directed toward easing her death, Mrs. W. was able to die quickly and pain-lessly, as she had hoped.

Mrs. W.'s overall clinical course spanned more than 15 years, none of which could have been reliably predicted at the outset. Therefore, the most important clinical and ethical elements might have been the commitment among health care providers, patient, and family to face an unknown future together, and to keep Mrs. W.'s interests and values at all times in the foreground of decision making. Physicians who make these commitments cannot be afraid of an aggressive fight for life that may temporarily be associated with considerable suffering, and they must also not be afraid of death as an important and inevitable part of the life cycle.

Advanced medical technology added meaningful years to Mrs. W.'s life. Yet that same technology could have made her dying a painful ordeal rather than a natural event if it had been used without restraint. Modern medicine is challenged to help people live longer and better, but also to die in ways that are both timely and dignified. This is no simple task. Illnesses can be unpredictable and variable, and people vary greatly with respect to what they consider dignified and meaningful. Therefore, working together over time, keeping the patient's values in the foreground, communicating carefully so that patients and families are able to grasp the meaning and impact of the decisions they are making, and facing hard end-of-life decisions together are all at the core of the clinical experience.

Overview

To better explore and understand the process of caring for patients and their families at the end of life, the chapters in this book are organized into three parts.

Part I focuses on Underlying Values and Assumptions, with particular emphasis on critical values that underlie the doctor–patient relationship and the process of joint decision making. Several key elements of medical humanism are explored in the context of clinical narratives about two patients for whom I cared who had near-death experiences. The chapter on partnership is illustrated with a clinical narrative I initially wrote for the *New England Journal of Medicine* about my end-of-life decision making with a patient named Diane. The article placed me in the center of the so-called right-to-die debate. I argue that the means by which Diane died were much less important than the enduring commitment between doctor, patient, and family throughout the patient's illness. Part I culminates in a discussion about nonabandonment, which I feel is the most fundamental value articulating the commitment dying patients and their families need from health care providers. The analyses presented focus more on the personalized treatment of those who come under the care of any health care provider than on the equally important challenges of improving systems of care or health care policy.

Part II shifts to The Medical Interview: A Critical Clinical Tool. Communication skills about end-of-life issues with patients and families are essential to excellent palliative care and informed decision making. Unfortunately, these skills are complex and poorly taught in comparison to other vital clinical skills. The chapters in Part II provide practical guidance for clinicians, patients, and families for conducting critical conversations around several difficult topics, including delivering bad news, discussing palliative care, making decisions when patients can no longer participate, and talking with patients who express a wish to die.

Conversations in any of these four domains involve delicate emotional, ethical, and personal issues around death and dying. In many cases, they are put off or even avoided all together, often with devastating consequences. When these discussions are not pursued with the depth and seriousness that they deserve, the result usually is a continuation of aggressive treatment, and a concomitant under-recognition and under-treatment of human suffering. If we are to give severely ill patients and families humane care and meaningful choices, clear communication skills about end-of-life issues and committed relationships over time must become core clinical skills.

Part III focuses on the Difficult Clinical and Ethical Issues faced by clinicians, patients, and families as a routine part of end-of-life care. Although physician-assisted suicide has received the bulk of public and professional attention, it is a relatively infrequent consideration. Most patients want to know that there is an escape if their suffering becomes intolerable, but few reach a point where assisted suicide is the only acceptable approach. Nevertheless, difficult choices abound toward the end of life, in part as a result of our medical successes. Many severely ill patients and their families and doctors face a series of value-laden decisions as death approaches, often without a clear road map other than the patient's values and the physician's knowledge and clinical experience.

Several clinical, ethical, and policy challenges within routine hospice and palliative care will be explored in the first chapter of this part. The next chapter describes the potential and limitations of the rule of double effect as a guide to end-of-life decision making. In the third chapter of Part III, last-resort options that have been proposed for responding to severe suffering will be compared in their clinical, ethical, and legal dimensions, and practical safeguards will be considered. Unfortunately, these "last-resort" measures are a frequent part of end-of-life care, so clinicians should learn to judiciously use at least some of them in the service of patients and families who find themselves without any desirable alternatives. The last chapter in this section will compare end-of-life care in the Netherlands, where euthanasia and assisted suicide are illegal but openly tolerated,° with that in the United States, where assisted dying is generally prohibited. To better understand commonalities and differences, underlying values, justifications, legal systems, and practice patterns in the two countries will be compared.

Tragically for our family, my brother died from complications of a bicycling accident as I was completing work on this book. Making end-of-life decisions on his behalf while grieving with enormous intensity has provided a reality check for the ideas presented in this book. In the Epilogue, I chronicle our experience as a family through my brother's devastating injury and death, and reflect on the process from the other side of the looking glass.

Throughout the book, I repeatedly return to the importance of committed relationships. When a person is dying, usually his or her relationships with family and friends are at the core of the endeavor. Because medical and palliative care issues frequently arise, clinicians also become vitally important participants in this caring process. Although most of my focus is on physicians, this is in part because they are paradoxically the most powerful yet least reliable members of the health care team. In many cases, nurses are the pivotal health care providers toward the end of life, spending more time at the bedside than other providers, and often showing the kinds of commitments that I am advocating.

° Legislation legalizing euthanasia and assisted suicide was recently passed by the Dutch legislature, and full legalization is anticipated in 2001.

All clinicians should aspire to treat their patients with the caring, intensity, and attention to detail that they would want for themselves or their loved ones, and make the commitment to see the process through to a patient's death. The skills, challenges, and aspirations of excellent palliative care are articulated throughout the three parts of this book—relieving pain and symptoms, and giving patients and their families the opportunity to achieve peaceful resolution, where possible and desired by the patient, at the end of life. However, this work also potentially involves addressing intractable and intolerable situations, depending on the course of the patient's illness.

My hope is that readers will learn more about what is possible at the end of life—both the potential for great meaning and personal connection, and also the possibility of devastation and disintegration. The task is both to promote the opportunities that dying presents for the patient and family where possible, and to respond to the destructive potential when necessary. Patients and families are counting on our responsiveness, creativity, and guidance as we face their uncertain future together.

References

1. Doyle D, Hanks GW, MacDonald N. *Oxford Textbook of Palliative Medicine*, 2nd ed. Oxford: Oxford University Press, 1998.
2. Rhymes J. Hospice care in America. *JAMA* 1990; 264:369–372.
3. Stoddard S. Hospice in the United States: An overview. *J Palliat Care* 1989; 5:10.

1

Same Old Seventeen-Dollar Lamps

I was a medical intern in 1976 when I met the Reverend, a fundamentalist African-American preacher. The Reverend had no faith in medical technology or its practitioners and had vowed never to enter a hospital. Life and death, in his opinion, should be left exclusively in God's hands. Until then, his strategy had worked well. However, at 85 years of age, the Reverend had embarked on the third 40 day fast of his life as a way to cleanse himself and become closer to God. Midway through this fast, he stopped drinking as well as eating. As he drifted into a deep coma, his parishioners became uncomfortable with what they were witnessing.

The church elders brought the Reverend to the hospital. Although they were acting against his express wishes, the elders could not bear to watch him die. If he recovered, they were willing to bear his disapproval. Together, faith and medicine might be more powerful than either could be separately.

The Reverend was brought to us neatly dressed in a starched shirt and pressed pants. Underneath, dry skin hung loosely from his shriveled body; his tongue looked like a sliver of dehydrated fruit. He was unresponsive, even to painful stimulation. His blood pressure was extremely low, his kidneys were failing, and his blood electrolytes were very abnormal. It was

This story was originally published in *Annals of Internal Medicine* 1999; 130:835–840.

possible that he would not survive. I felt uncertain about imposing treatment against the Reverend's will, but given the reversibility of his condition, we reassured ourselves that his prestated wishes might not apply to this particular circumstance.

We vigorously replenished his fluids and gradually corrected his electrolytes, trying to avoid damage to his severely dehydrated brain. We invaded his body with needles and catheters, drawing his blood every few hours to monitor the changes. When he developed brisk gastrointestinal bleeding, we gave him several transfusions. We received consent from the church elders for major procedures and pushed forward without self-reflection in a vigorous fight to save his life. Over the next five days, his blood pressure and kidney function began to improve, but he remained unresponsive.

We decided to discuss the Reverend's case at Professor's Rounds. Ten residents and students and our professor surrounded his bed as I began my ritualized presentation. "Reverend A. is an 85 year-old man who was brought to the hospital in the middle of a 40 day fast, profoundly dehydrated after drinking no fluids. His medical history was unremarkable. He has completed two previous fasts without incident. . . ." As I proceeded with his medical history, I noticed that the Reverend's eyes were open. His gaze had previously been vacant and disconnected, but now a spark was in his eyes, and he seemed to be looking directly at me.

"Reverend, how are you feeling? Can you hear me?" I paused, anxious about breaking from the usual format of the teaching rounds.

The Reverend stirred, looked around the room, and began: "God damn you! What in hell do you think you are doing to me? You sons of bitches! . . ." On and on the Reverend ranted, raged, and cursed. No one knew what to say or how to respond. Bathed in sweat, our ordinarily resourceful professor finally suggested that we leave the room. The Reverend's parishioners took over and quietly calmed and supported their leader.

We returned to the classroom, barely acknowledging what had just happened. The Reverend's recovery was attributed to our medical interventions, and the "outburst" was attributed to delirium. We spent the next hour discussing his complex fluid and electrolyte abnormalities.

During the next two weeks, the Reverend discussed his near-death experience with us as he recovered. He was thankful to his parishioners for bringing him to the hospital. Although he appreciated our medical efforts to save his life, the Reverend attributed his recovery to God's will. He described his time while comatose in glowing terms. He had "seen the other side, and it was beautiful." He was not sure at first whether he wanted to return to this life. His time in the hospital had been God's way of letting him know that he had nothing to fear about death, and his ministry would be immeasurably enriched and informed by his experience.

For us, caring for the Reverend reinforced much of what was appealing in medicine. We believed that we had defeated death with medical technology. The Reverend left the hospital fully restored. Although his report about the "other side" was never thought to be an appropriate topic for our formal medical education, we learned that death might not be as frightening as we thought. The Reverend's encounter with death seemed powerfully reassuring to us, especially with regard to other, less fortunate patients. The Reverend's vision took some of the sting out of the medical battles we lost.

In my subsequent 20 years of practice, I have cared for many persons who have a clear vision about an afterlife, and a few who have had near-death experiences. The diversity of these experiences astonishes me; the clarity with which some patients talk about them is one of the great treasures of working with the dying. I do not have a simple system for understanding or predicting these experiences. Some patients with a peaceful notion of an afterlife fight death to the bitter end, and others with little outward sense of spirituality approach death with calm acceptance. The last chapter of our lives is written in part by our choices and values, but it is also determined by arbitrary and capricious forces. Part of our job as healers is to help patients decide what remains to be accomplished within the constraints of their illness and to help them respond creatively to forces and events that are out of their personal control.

With this in mind, I cared for Mrs. M., who also had had a near-death experience. She had successfully overcome alcoholism, breast cancer, and depression during the 15 years we worked together. Mrs. M. and her husband divorced when their children were very young, and she raised two daughters as a single mother, working two jobs through their entire childhood. Having witnessed firsthand the ravages of heavy drinking, Mrs. M.'s daughters were wary of their mother. They came to her side briefly when she had surgery for breast cancer and then left town at the first opportunity. Mrs. M. worked hard as an executive secretary but had no social life outside of work. She liked nothing better than to go home to a good book, sip manhattans, and smoke cigarettes. She was raised a Roman Catholic, but over the years she became alienated from the church.

Our initial meetings were exclusively medical in focus, but over several years I got a glimpse of her personal life. She eventually stopped drinking after being confronted by her daughters. She then regularly attended Alcoholics Anonymous and maintained sobriety. Although she was content, she remained isolated, with little joy except the escape she found in reading fiction. I eventually convinced her to try antidepressant medications, which helped her mood considerably. Still, outside of her medical visits she remained alone most of the time. I came to respect her quiet vigilance and dignity. We gradually became friends.

Several years later, Mrs. M. developed abdominal pain that led to a diagnosis of metastatic adenocarcinoma. After exploring all of the medical options, including experimental therapy, Mrs. M. chose a hospice approach. She did not want to die, but she had no desire to incur additional suffering in a futile medical battle. She had suffered enough. Although her prognosis was less than six months, she initially did not qualify for a home hospice program because she did not have a primary caregiver. I convinced her to share the dilemma with her daughters, and fortunately they volunteered to help care for their mother in a home hospice program.

Mrs. M. experienced the kind of personal growth that one hopes for at the end of life. She had healing contact with her daughters, who forgave her for past hurts. They expressed love and appreciation for the hard work, caring, and commitment it took to raise them as a single parent. Mrs. M. shared stories of her own childhood as an immigrant, which made her struggles as a parent more understandable. She met with her parish priest and worked through some of her anger at God and the church for abandoning her during her years of drinking and alienation. The last chapter of Mrs. M.'s life was filled with meaningful contact, but it was not all hard work: There were laughs, card games, and a few good books she had yet to read.

Mrs. M.'s pain was easily controlled. As death approached, she gradually stopped eating and drinking. Mrs. M., her family, and I had several long talks about how this was a natural part of dying that was relatively free of suffering. We would keep her mouth moist and follow her lead by providing sips of liquids and small amounts of her favorite foods as she wished. Mrs. M. was peaceful about her death. Her life had come together in her last months more than she had ever dreamed was possible. Mrs. M. did not have a clear vision of an afterlife, and she had no fantasies of being reunited with her deceased parents or her ex-husband in the next life. In fact, she quipped, such a fate would be worse than death.

As she slipped into a coma, her family sat at the bedside in a peaceful vigil. They wanted reassurance that their mother was not starving to death. Mrs. M. remained quietly unresponsive for five days as the family waited. It had been a meaningful process for them, and they had done a good job. Dying was not nearly as frightening as it had once seemed.

On day six, I got a phone call. Mrs. M. seemed to be reawakening. She had opened her eyes and was asking for sips of water. What was going on? What should they do? Where had she been? Would I please come out and visit? As I prepared myself to see Mrs. M., I too was filled with questions that only she could answer. Had she had a near-death experience that I could learn from? Had she chosen to come back because she was not "ready" or because of some unfinished business? Does one view these events medically or spiritually? I wasn't sure I knew the right questions, but I did have a desire to learn from her experience and help make sense out of what had happened.

Mrs. M. seemed very weak, but her eyes were fully alive.

"Welcome back," I said.

She smiled and said, "Thanks."

"How are you feeling?" I asked.

"Not bad," she answered.

"What was it like?" I queried.

"It was all very dark and empty. No thought, no people, no colors. Just blackness. It was not unpleasant. In fact, it was reasonably peaceful. And no sense of time. I remember a light, kind of hazy at first. [*Light? What light? I wondered.*] Then the light became brighter and clearer, and it dawned on me that it was those same old seventeen-dollar lamps across the room on the mantel that I saw before I went to sleep! I was glad to see my daughters but disappointed to still be here."

She laughed as she told me this story. Yet there were tears in our eyes: sadness about life's unfairness and perhaps about a vision—a light—that wasn't. I told her I was glad that she would get a little more time and that we would help her make the most of it. Her daughters wanted to know what was going on; I responded that these processes sometimes have unusual twists. Our job at this time was to go with the flow of what was happening and to make sure that all that needed to be said was said.

Mrs. M. died quietly about 48 hours later. How and why she awoke after such a long and seemingly deep sleep remains a mystery to me. I can concoct some explanations, but in the final analysis, we don't know. I had to laugh at the way I had reacted as she told her story of "embracing the light." I had been hanging on every word, hoping for a glimpse of the unknown and unknowable. Therein lies the beauty and the mystery of this work, and the thing that keeps us coming back.

2

Humanistic End-of-Life Care

The Reverend and Mrs. M. both undertook complicated medical journeys with positive outcomes. The Reverend was fortunate to recover fully and return to preaching, enriched by a reaffirming medical and spiritual experience. Mrs. M. had a peaceful death, preceded by a time of healing and coming together for her and her daughters. Both cases, however, illustrate how overly simplistic notions of humanism and ethics will not easily withstand the realities patients and their families face. How could we justify overriding the Reverend's clearly articulated advance directive that under no circumstances should he go to a hospital or undergo medical treatment? On the other hand, how could we not treat the Reverend, since his illness was not only reversible but to a large extent self-imposed by a religious ritual gone awry? Taking the Reverend's advance directive at face value, without trying to understand how it applied to his specific circumstances, could have resulted in a premature death. Yet overriding an advance directive simply because a patient might survive with our potent medical interventions can undermine an individual's integrity as a person and prolong unwanted suffering, more akin to assault and battery than humane treatment. How, then, do we want the medical profession to proceed in conditions of considerable moral and clinical uncertainty, which is the rule in medicine rather than the exception?

I have struggled to come up with a working definition of humanism in medicine. The *Oxford English Dictionary* defines it as "a doctrine, attitude, or way of life centered on human interests or values; a philosophy . . . that stresses an individual's dignity and worth and capacity for self-realization through reason."[1] In medicine, humanism becomes manifest through caring relationships between health care providers, patients, and their families. A "patient-centered" approach focuses on the patient as the subject of care, emphasizing the centrality of the patient's values as well as his or her body and soul as the recipient of care.[2,3] Others have preferred conceptualizing a "relationship-centered" approach, underscoring the dynamic reciprocal interplay among doctor, patient, family, and society.[4] Though final decisions ultimately must flow from patients and their representatives, this model may better serve human beings struggling with severe illness by keeping them connected with their families and with health care providers.

Putting a humanistic approach into practice in the modern medical environment is no simple matter, for it requires a combination of competencies in multiple medical domains, as well as relationship-centered skills and values. A good distillation of this approach emerged in a conversation I had with a colleague friend. How committed would we be in the care of a patient with whom we had a deep personal bond, or perhaps with a close colleague, friend, or family member? In this circumstance, if a treatment existed that would be helpful in treating disease or relieving suffering, we would go the extra mile or 100 miles to learn about it and gain access to it. If the patient began to experience terrible suffering prior to death, we would assiduously work with him or her until it was relieved. No potentially helpful intervention would be categorically excluded in this search. As Francis Peabody put it, "The secret in the care of the patient is to care about the patient."[5] Of course, it is easier to do this when one instinctively feels a strong emotional bond with a patient, and harder to do it with a patient who is not well known or is very different culturally or experientially. Nevertheless, that is the challenge of the humanistic physician.

My bond with Mrs. M. evolved over many years of working together, as she faced and overcame depression, breast cancer, and alcoholism. Partly as a result of this shared experience, we trusted each other to be perfectly frank with respect to how we saw her situation. With the Reverend, there was no prior relationship. What we knew about him led us to believe that when and if he awakened, he would probably reject our efforts. We could easily have relied on a simplistic notion of autonomy, and not treated his ailments aggressively because of his prior statements about not wanting medical intervention of any kind. But if we were to treat him as we would a member of our own family, we had to think carefully about the specifics of his medical situation and his personal values. His dehydration and kidney failure had a good chance of being

TABLE 2–1. Critical Dimensions of Humanistic Care

Competence
  Medical, palliative care
  Ethical
  Cultural
Communication skills
Empathic imagination
Self-awareness
Healing
Partnership
Nonabandonment

reversible. Yet in order to adequately treat him, we would have to invade his body with multiple blood tests, tubes in his stomach and urinary bladder, possibly even dialysis or mechanical ventilation. In considering his values, we knew that he respected life tremendously but that he also had little use for medical technology. His intention in initiating the fast was to experience a spiritual cleansing, but in no way did he intend to end his life. Along with the parishioners who were representing him, we struggled to comprehend what the Reverend would want us to do, and we reached the tentative conclusion that he would want to proceed with medical intervention as long as there was a good chance of recovery. Our knowledge about his wishes was uncertain, so one hopes we would have had the courage to rethink our decision had his clinical situation and prognosis worsened.

Several elements of humanistic care stand out in these two cases. The aspects of care that I have chosen to cover in this chapter are competence (medical, palliative care, ethical, cultural), communication skills, empathic imagination, self-awareness, and healing. Partnership and nonabandonment, which I see as critical additional elements, will be explored in subsequent chapters.

Competence

A caring, humanistic physician who is not competent in the biomedical aspects of medicine would not be of great use to a patient facing severe illness. The Reverend and his parishioners needed someone to make an accurate assessment of his medical condition, including his potential for full recovery or survival with significant limitations, and the likelihood of death. Once we decided to move forward with aggressive treatment, he needed skilled medical practitioners to use modern medical treatments to give him the best chance of recovery. His recovery depended on careful attention to all of the details of his metabolic state. Had the Reverend been severely chronically ill before the fast, his potential for full recovery would have been considerably less, perhaps leading to a different decision about the proper course of action. Thus, competence is needed both in assessing prognosis and treatment options, and then in skillfully executing the path chosen.

When Mrs. M. decided that she did not want aggressive treatment for her stomach cancer, she needed to learn about the efficacy of the medical intervention she was forgoing. If, for example, she had lymphoma, then her chances for long-term survival and even cure with treatment would have been good. Adenocarcinoma of the stomach, however, has a poor prognosis with or without aggressive treatment. Still, in treating her as one would a family member, the clinician should explore whether any promising experimental therapy is on the horizon, and all potentially effective interventions can be considered.

In addition to competence at treating medical diseases, clinicians caring for severely ill patients must have competence in palliative care. This means effectively managing pain and other symptoms,[6] as well as talking with patients about their hopes and fears and their possible death. In Mrs. M.'s case, these issues were relevant whether she chose intensive disease-directed treatment or entered a hospice program where the main goal is palliation. Mrs. M.'s initial fear was pain, and I was able to reassure her that we could help her manage almost all kinds of pain, and that we could give her very large doses of opioids if they were needed. Then we began to explore what she still needed to accomplish given her limited life span. She wanted to devote most of her remaining time and energy to reconnecting with her daughters. Mrs. M. hoped that she and her daughters could achieve a deeper understanding of one another, forgiveness for not being there for each other in the past, and deep expressions of love and thanks. Had she not accepted that she was dying, this opportunity for such connection and closure might have been lost.

In addition to medical and palliative care competencies, these cases illustrate the importance of ethical competence. Mrs. M. was within her rights in turning down aggressive medical therapy directed at her gastric cancer, as well as in choosing not to receive cardiopulmonary resuscitation. Offering her as much opioid medication as she needed in the future to control her pain is well within accepted medical practice, even in doses that might be sedating.[7] Since death would be foreseen as a potential side effect and not the intention of this intervention, such treatment could be justified according to the rule of double effect, which has become a cornerstone of medical ethics in the United States. As we will see in the next chapter, had Mrs. M. requested medication that could be taken as an overdose should her suffering become overwhelming in the future, she would have asked her physician to enter an ethical and legal gray zone. Ideally, humanistic physicians will use the same standards with their patients that they would use with their own family or close friends. Of course, what we would do in exceptional circumstances to help people who come under our care is a question separate from whether legalizing such practices is good public policy.

What about the Reverend's case from an ethical perspective? Unfortunately, the Reverend initially could not speak for himself. Although he had no formal living will or health care proxy, he had made his wishes and values clear to his parishioners. The challenge of substituted judgment is to make the decision as the Reverend would, given his values and his current clinical circumstances. The Quinlan court posed the correct question: If [the Reverend] could wake up for 10 minutes and understand his situation completely, what would [he] tell you to do?[8] As is often the case, we could not discern with certainty what the Reverend would tell us under such circumstances. Clearly he would submit to God's will, but did God's will include aggressive medical intervention? It seemed likely that if he could fully recover, he would want our interventions. It was also possible that we would save his body but significantly injure his 85 year-old brain in the process. Given this uncertainty, we were not sure what he would tell us to do, so we erred on the side of fighting for his survival. If the outcome was less than favorable, we would work with the parishioners to pick up the pieces of his life, again guided by the Reverend's values as much as possible.

With the Reverend, we were also crossing a substantial cultural and spiritual divide. Although health care practitioners cannot be expert at knowing the nuances of all cultures, races, and religions, they must be aware when cultural differences exist, and then know how to explore them.[9-11] For example, we now know that cultural and racial biases influence access to treatments for lung cancer[12] as well as cardiac catheterization rates.[13] Any lack of trust between African-American patients and Caucasian physicians is based in part on such presumably unconscious biased behavior, as well as more egregious past incidents.[14]

Furthermore, physicians as a group tend to be nonreligious by comparison with patients.[15-18] The Reverend had strong Christian fundamentalist beliefs that were highly relevant to his care but likely to be somewhat alien to many on the health care team. The Reverend would be much more likely to look to God for guidance than to his medical providers. Physicians and other health care providers tend to put much more of their faith in the power of medical science to thwart death and disease. Clinicians must be aware of how their own priorities, beliefs, and values may conflict with those of their patients—and perhaps determine the types of care that they offer. They must also try as best they can to explore the cultural and spiritual dimensions of a patient's life so they can enrich the caring process rather than hamper it.

We identified the Reverend's church elders as his chief advocates, and met with them on a regular basis. Once we achieved a consensus about trying aggressive treatment, we apprised the elders of the Reverend's medical progress each day. We also inquired about any concerns or observations they might have, keeping in mind that their strong faith would be an especially important resource should his clinical course not turn out well. We were aware that his congregation would help support and sustain him if he emerged in less than optimal shape either physically or mentally. When the Reverend awoke in a strange environment during Professor's Rounds, his parishioners were there to comfort him and help him make sense of what had happened. After he had recovered, the Reverend had no qualms about our having aggressively intervened.

Communication

Communication skills are at the core of humane medicine. Good communication permits patients and families to make decisions that reflect the complexity of clinical medicine as well as their personal values and preferences. When Mrs. M. was faced with making a decision about how to approach her newly diagnosed stomach cancer, she needed information about this type of cancer: its natural history, and how it usually responds to medical treatment. After she learned that the prognosis was not favorable with or without medical treatment, it was incumbent on me, as her physician, to learn about her values and priorities in light of this new information. Was she willing to risk increased suffering during her final days, weeks, or months in order to fight her disease with experimental therapy? Or would she rather avoid additional iatrogenic suffering and spend as much time as possible at home with her family? By listening carefully to her preferences and the personal experiences that underlay her values and priorities, I learned that Mrs. M. wanted to minimize suffering and maximize her quality of life for the time that remained.

Had she wanted to fight for life with anything that might work, even if it involved additional suffering, then we would have had to more fully explore experimental medical therapy. These treatments *could* work (they had not been shown not to work), though the chances for prolonged survival in this particular disease were probably less than 1%. Why not try it at least? To be fully informed, a patient and family would have to learn what happens to the other 99%. Chemotherapy, radiation, and surgery were combined in the experimental protocol—interventions associated with considerable added suffering. Such added hardship might be worth it if one were in the 1% that survived, but it would seem a harsh way to treat a person if she were in the 99% who don't. Some patients would find such a fight against disease and death critical to them as persons. For example, some patients who have been prisoners of war and survived against all odds simply cannot imagine giving in to illness and death no matter how poor the odds. Others might draw the opposite conclusion from the same experience: that they have already suffered so much that it would be meaningless to submit to the added futile suffering that would come from medical intervention.

Some patients will make different decisions depending on how the information is framed. "There is a 1% chance the treatment could work!" and "There is a 99% chance that the treatment won't work" are opposite sides of the same coin. To be fully informed, the patient needs to learn about what happens to both the 1% and the 99%, ideally spending time exploring such information in depth.[19]

The physician should not be a passive agent whose job is to simply provide "options" from which the patient must choose.[20] Informing the patient about the range of possibilities is an important starting point, but then the physician must use his or her knowledge and experience to help the patient make the best decision given the patient's values and clinical situation. With Mrs. M., the decision-making process was relatively easy, since we both understood that experimental treatments were toxic and invasive (chemotherapy, radiation, and surgery), and the odds of their working were remote. Had she wanted to pursue aggressive experimental therapy, we would have had to have serious discussions wherein I would become informed about how she saw the choices and she would become informed about how I saw them. I would support her choice once I fully understood it, as long as I believed that she was fully informed, but neither of us would be well served by being passive or neutral in these discussions.

The second section of this book is devoted to critical communication issues, including the delivery of bad news, how to discuss palliative care with patients who can communicate for themselves and those who cannot, and how to respond to those who express a wish to die. The exploration of these domains will illustrate humane end-of-life care, including joint decision making and maintaining relationships that are both caring and informative among health care providers, patients, and families. Communication about complex end-of-life issues is one of the weakest links in our efforts to improve care and choices at this phase of life, yet it remains pivotal in allowing patients and families to make the most of the end of their lives. Treating patients and their families as you would like your own family members and friends to be treated is a tough standard, for it requires genuinely caring about the outcome and using both medical and palliative care systems in an intensely personal and individualized way. Given the inherent limits imposed by one's illness, why not treat our patients exactly as we would want to be treated ourselves, and communicate with them as clearly, personally, and humanely as possible?

Empathic Imagination

Empathy is defined as the ability to place oneself within the lived experience of another—in simple terms, to walk in another's shoes.[21] To experience empathy, one must have a combination of excellent interviewing skills and a vivid ability to imagine both the emotional and cognitive experiences of another. As one hears about an individual's particular story of illness, and listens to it with an open mind and an open heart, one begins to "get a feel" for the patient's inner experience. This feel may be vague and imprecise initially, but it can be clarified by encouraging the patient to give a detailed account of the experience. The next step is to try to identify with the experience, using one's own human experience and imagination as well as what is known about the patient. Sometimes the patient's experience can be acknowledged (*"That must have been terrifying for you"*) or validated (*"Anyone who had experienced such a shock would have been frightened"*). The deeper understanding of the patient's experience that emanates from the patient's responses to these statements helps a physician or other care provider build empathy.[22,23]

Opponents of more open access to physician-assisted death as a last resort have criticized advocates as having a "failure of imagination" about the opportunity for meaning and growth at the end of life.[24] Many practitioners, patients, and family members do indeed lack a vision about the opportunity for self-fulfillment and human connection that is sometimes possible at the end of life. However, many patients and families criticize opponents of physician-assisted death for a lack of imagination in a different realm. Practitioners must also try to understand and explore the suffering that might drive a seriously ill patient to contemplate ending his or her life.[25] Only after fully exploring and empathically imagining the patient's circumstances can one begin to treat the patient as a loved one and to imagine options or approaches that are congruent with the patient's values and respectful of him or her as a person.

Whereas empathy involves feeling with or feeling as the patient, sympathy involves a feeling of sorrow for the patient. Sympathy occurs when the physician acknowledges the patient's loss, but it is marked by the expresser staying on a different (and usually superior) plane than the patient. I might "feel sorry for you" (about your condition, illness, or loss), but I don't necessarily understand or appreciate your feelings or experience. Empathy, on the other hand, is having a strong identification with what the patient is feeling, which allows for much greater emotional and existential proximity. This vantage point may allow the physician to contemplate decisions more as the patient would make them. It reintroduces the subjective into medicine, and stops the practice of pretending that decisions can be based exclusively on an "objective" probabilistic analysis.

When a physician begins to truly enter the patient's world, including its more difficult aspects, both physician and patient experience a sense of connection.[26] There may be physiologic correlates, such as tearing when a patient is crying or experiencing goose bumps when the patient is frightened, allowing the clinician to understand that his or her emotions and cognition are in sync with the patient's. Even if there is no simple way to address or resolve the patient's dilemma, at least the patient is no longer alone with his or her thoughts and feelings. Frequently, the feeling of connection enhances the clinician's commitment to work with the patient in a way that is based squarely on the patient's experience and values rather than those of the physician.

How might empathy and imagination be realized with Mrs. M. or the Reverend? Let us begin with Mrs. M., whose inner life began to take on depth and shape for me when I heard about her struggles to raise two children as a single mother, and about how she finally found the courage to take on and eventually overcome her alcohol addiction. After initially being diagnosed with stomach cancer, Mrs. M. stated that she had "suffered enough." One could not respond empathically to this statement without having some understanding of her past suffering. Had I not known her life story, I might have asked her to tell me more about how she had suffered in the past. As her story unfolds, and the interviewer begins to get a more complete picture of her as a person, it is much easier to join with her in making decisions consistent with her values. For Mrs. M., who was quite isolated at first, there were no other friends or family who understood enough about her to appreciate what she was going through.

Having heard that she had deep regret about her relationship with her daughters, and knowing her desire for some kind of forgiveness and restitution, I was able to help Mrs. M. ask her daughters to participate in her terminal care. This approach was so much more meaningful than experimental therapy would have been for Mrs. M., yet for another patient, with a different life experience, the opposite may have been true. As Mrs. M. gradually stopped eating and drinking, and slipped into a coma, I understood enough about her goals and wishes to be clearly communicate to her daughters that she would not want artificial feeding or hydration. I was then able to reassure them that they had already given her the most precious gift possible—their loving presence and forgiveness.

How might empathy and imagination have worked with the Reverend? Here the task was more formidable, for not only were there substantial cultural differences, but the Reverend could not speak for himself. To make matters more complex, we were initially told that the Reverend had never wanted to be taken to the hospital in the first place. Yet as we began to understand the Reverend's story, we learned that the goal of his fast was to become closer to God, and to use the fruits of that experience to enrich his ministry in this life. We heard nothing about his being prepared for death, or even considering that such a ritual might make death a possibility. His profound dehydration was completely unanticipated. Therefore, our task was to take what we could learn, join with those parishioners who knew him best, and try to empathically imagine what he would want us to do. Although we might have been wrong, our collective imagination suggested that aggressive treatment would have been his wish under these circumstances.

When patients cannot speak for themselves, they depend on us to use what is known about their values and clinical condition, and to make decisions as we believe they would under the circumstances. The skills needed here are a combination of good detective work about the person's values and experience, and a skilled clinical assessment of the disease process, including its prognosis with and without treatment, followed finally by using one's empathic imagination to make a decision as the patient would. The Reverend confirmed that we made the right decision; he was glad that God gave us the wisdom to intervene on his behalf.

This is not to say we should always err on the side of aggressive treatment when there is any uncertainty, for there is never 100 percent certainty about a person's wishes when it comes to substituted judgment. Nevertheless, we must use what is known about the patient to make the best decision possible, using his or her values rather than our own. A combination of empathic imagination and consensus building by those who care about the patient is the best possible guide during these difficult times.[27]

Self-Awareness

If one is to engage with patients and their families in this intensely personal way, considerable self-awareness is required. At the simplest level, one may confuse one's own feelings and values with those of the patient. The question of what we ourselves would do in the patient's circumstances is an important one, but it speaks to our own values and experience, not the patient's. Similarly, the sadness or anger that a clinician may feel when interacting with a patient may be a clue to how the patient is feeling, but it may also reflect the physician's own emotional state or personal reaction to the patient rather than any true empathic understanding.

Sorting out feelings and values takes considerable practice, and improves with training and repetition.[28] Unfortunately, most physicians are given little encouragement or training in looking inside themselves and exploring potential sources of strong reactions and identifications. In fact, there may frequently be a conspiracy to suppress such reactions, in the belief that they should not exist in a "professional" physician–patient relationship. Yet these explorations are an important part of the training and evolution of a humanistic physician.

Many clinicians recognize the feelings and reactions of others with much greater clarity than they do in themselves.[29] They have frequently been care-takers within their own families from an early age, suppressing their own emotional growth and self-awareness in the interest of serving others. At first blush, this may seem to enhance clinicians' capacities for understanding of and empathy for their patients. On the other hand, more complex feelings of resent-ment and anger may emerge, and these physicians may be able to look only to the patient and not to themselves for explanations about what they are experiencing.[28,30] A truly self-aware clinician will be able to determine if the source of a strong reaction is the clinician him- or herself, the patient, or the interaction of the two.

Let us see how self-awareness might affect the care of the Reverend and Mrs. M. I encountered the Reverend early in my training, when I was just beginning to come to grips with the dark side of medicine's ability to simulta-neously prolong life and prolong dying. As members of the hospital healthcare team, we were repeatedly encountering frail patients who were extremely ill and appeared to be dying, and we were blindly fighting against death using all available medical technology. Being a medical intern, I was a foot soldier in this monolithic and sometimes futile battle. At its most extreme, we would electri-cally shock the heart repeatedly, crush the chest, and invade all parts of the bodies of frail, elderly, dying patients. The senior physicians who were order-ing this invasion were nowhere to be found as these interventions were imple-mented. At an emotional level, it felt at times as if we were torturing dying people up to and including the moment of their death.

There were a few victories, as with the Reverend, but the failures and added suffering seemed disproportionately high. The lack of clarity surrounding the goals of treatment was usually not part of the medical dialogue. In fact, one's devotion to the practice of medicine might be called into question if one raised doubts about the preferred approach. Perhaps my hesitance meant that I was not a dedicated enough professional. Perhaps others who had more clarity of purpose would be more able to help patients and their families. Yet some patients and their families were very reluctant about what they were going through, did not know how to stop the process, and mainly wanted relief from their suffering. For them, we were clearly doing more harm than good.

In the midst of this confusion, and in a world in which such conflict was almost never openly explored, how were we to address the Reverend's dilemma? The dominant medical ethos of the day was unequivocally to treat an underlying illness that had a substantial chance of being reversible. Although his age and his profound degree of dehydration and kidney failure made the odds of his recovery around 50%, this would be more than enough to warrant our proceeding. Conversely, the principle of substituted judgment suggested that we respect the patient's autonomy by avoiding any medical interventions—even those that would likely be effective.

My initial personal reaction was one of ambivalence. The Reverend had a better chance than most of recovery, but what if he only partially recovered? What if his body recovered but his mind did not? If we started this process, did it mean that he was consenting to any and all medical interventions no matter how invasive—and even if his condition deteriorated? On the other side of the coin, I was not at all sure what the Reverend would want us to do under these circumstances. The information we had about his wishes was too superficial to warrant nontreatment under these unique circumstances. Furthermore, his parishioners were supporting the idea of a treatment trial to see if his condition could be reversed. If he deteriorated, we could rethink our strategy. The challenge for the self-aware physician was to think through all of the potential conflicting forces and try to make the decision the Reverend would if he could speak for himself.

In the Reverend's case, we made the right decision. This was not simply because he survived and walked out of the hospital (we had resuscitated some severely ill patients against their will who were very distressed to have survived), but rather that he appreciated our efforts and believed that we had done the right thing. I want to believe that we struggled to represent the Reverend's will in making these decisions, but I also remember the pressure to aggressively treat all patients in those days. Therefore, we may have done the right thing for the wrong reasons. Nevertheless, we took joy in this success, and in the experience of helping to bring the Reverend back from the dead.

The Reverend's experience of "the other side" was also food for thought and reflection, though it was a topic that was considered "nonmedical." To be considered self-aware, a physician must grapple with the meaning of life and death, including the possibility of life after death, and therefore should become a student of such subjective experiences.

What about Mrs. M.? When she was struggling with alcoholism and depression early on in our relationship, I had to contemplate my own impatience and irritation with her. This did not stem from anything she said or did, but rather from the ravages that alcoholism has inflicted on my own family. I have learned more about my own family background in this regard, and I understand that my anger when confronting an alcoholic patient usually has less to do with that person than with my own personal issues. These reactions had to be put in perspective before I could begin to see Mrs. M.'s strengths and unique characteristics as a person. By the time she was diagnosed with stomach cancer, I had moved well beyond seeing her as an "alcoholic," and instead knew her as a single mother of two grown children, as a person who loved reading and knitting, as someone who had taken to drink in the past to self-medicate for depression and loneliness, and as an employee who had worked extremely diligently at her job as an executive secretary for more than 30 years. From this vantage point, I saw her as someone whose medical outcome was extremely important to me. Had we faced these decisions as strangers, particularly if she were still drinking heavily at the time, I would have had to work much harder to see her clearly as a person, and to personally care about what happened to her. Yet that would have been my challenge.

Healing

Healing is defined in a traditional biomedical setting in terms of curing patients of their diseases. Because of the prevalence of chronic diseases that cannot be cured, the definition has been expanded to include helping patients adjust to chronic disease and disability. Inevitably, this requires that patients be considered as persons with their own families and their own social and cultural contexts. Still, a central element of the healer's job is to fight alongside a patient for prolongation of life, to help the patient and family adjust to the consequences of chronic illness and of the medical treatment process. Death is usually considered to be a medical failure in this model—something to be fought off using all of medicine's resources, even if the treatment engenders additional suffering.

Patients who are dying need a broader model of healing—one that includes death as a natural and inevitable part of the life cycle. Modern medicine has been remarkably successful in prolonging life by developing treatments for many of the potentially fatal diseases that afflict human beings. But each success has created a new set of challenges. The last chapter of our lives is now likely to be filled with a progressive loss of independence and an increase in suffering and medical dependence.[31,32] We are far more likely to die in a hospital or nursing home than in our own home.[31] Instead of being surrounded by loved ones for our last hours or days, we may be tied to machines in a vain attempt to rescue us from inevitable death. It is as rare to find a "natural life" among those of advanced age as it is to find a "natural death." Life prolongation is usually desirable, but if life becomes dominated by suffering that can end only in death, then what is being prolonged is suffering and dying, and that is frequently not good.

Paradoxically, because of medicine's successes in extending life almost indefinitely, patients, families, and clinicians are today frequently faced with vexing questions about when to stop treatment, or whether to treat the next complication. Thus, we in medicine make life-and-death decisions on a daily basis; this is frequently done with family members rather than the patient, because so many patients eventually lose the capacity to participate in decision making due to the ravages of terminal illnesses. Here the healing task shifts from prolonging life at all costs to relieving suffering. One of the most terrifying aspects of dying in the modern era is the possibility of personal disintegration—existentially and personally falling apart before death.[33]

Dying can be a time of personal growth to find new meaning and connection in life, especially if the dying person is aware that death is near.[24,34] For the person who defined him- or herself in terms of physical abilities or job productivity, there is inevitable psychic pain as one gives up these abilities. There may also be an opportunity to spend time and energy on activities that perhaps had been shortchanged in the past, such as being with family and friends, exploring the meaning of one's life, writing, or reading. Many have come to believe that being diagnosed with a severe, terminal illness allowed for some of the best moments in their lives, because they gave themselves permission to experience vulnerability and personal connection with friends, family, or a higher power that had not been possible before.

Although we should promote and encourage such growth, not everyone can experience it. Some may experience it for a time, but then become challenged by their disease in ways that are personally threatening.[35] Sometimes the meaning that is unearthed in the dying process is subsequently undermined as death approaches, especially when the last phase of life is accompanied by severe suffering or personal disintegration. This brings up two additional essential elements of a healing relationship: partnership and nonabandonment. These concepts will be explored in depth in subsequent chapters. They reflect a commitment by a clinician to face the unknown together with his or her patient and family. A healing relationship entails both a caring commitment and a willingness to continue to problem-solve as the patient's clinical course unfolds. Let us review how this commitment worked with the Reverend and Mrs. M., and how it might have been challenged if their clinical course took different turns. In the next chapter, we will further illustrate these concepts by presenting the story of Diane.

We initially took a risk in treating the Reverend's illness despite his prior statements that suggested he did not want such medical intervention. Two underlying clinical elements were critical. First, the illness he had was reasonably likely to be reversible. Second, his illness was unintentionally self-inflicted, and therefore not part of any natural disease process. Both of these elements were important to the parish elders who were speaking on behalf of the Reverend. The biggest risk in all of our eyes was that this man's body would survive but his mind, which had been so clear prior to this illness, would not. The church elders believed that the Reverend would not want to be kept alive if he could not preach or counsel, activities that had been central to him for all of his adult life.

The Reverend was very lucky. His body fully recovered, as did his mind and spirit. In fact, his religious beliefs were only reinforced by his vision while he was near death, and his antagonism toward organized medicine was tempered to some degree by his reconceptualizing it as an agent of God.

Imagine for a moment that the Reverend had only partially survived. His kidneys returned to normal, but he had a stroke while he was severely ill, leaving him unable to walk, talk, or swallow. Here we would have had even tougher issues to face, including second-guessing the wisdom of initially over-riding his wishes not to be brought to the hospital. His parishioners would def-initely not have abandoned him, but could they have provided the 24 hour care and supervision that he would have needed? If we determined that he could not swallow food without risking getting it into his lungs, should we put in a feeding tube to provide artificial hydration and nutrition? What if he was alert but could not speak or consistently communicate? If he could have understood his situation, what would *he* have told us to do? If we believed that he would not want a feeding tube, could his parishioners and health care providers have tolerated sitting at his bedside as he gradually again became dehydrated and went back into kidney failure? Would the Reverend rather have died peacefully of the complications of his stroke at that time, or should we have provided artificial hydration and nutrition for a few months to see how he adjusted to his disability? Easy answers to these questions would have been unavailable. Yet the Reverend and his parishioners would have had to face these decisions had his illness gone another way, and they would have been better prepared to do so with a medical partner who was unequivocally committed to his well-being. Healing under such adverse circumstances would mean keeping the Reverend's personhood and values, as interpreted by his church elders, in mind at all times.

When Mrs. M. was diagnosed with stomach cancer, she was willing to let nature take its course, even though that course inevitably ended in her death. She wanted her pain and symptoms to be relieved, but she also hoped to have the opportunity to settle personal affairs with her daughters before she died. Dying presented an opportunity for a different kind of healing for Mrs. M., for she was able to come together with her daughters to give and receive forgive-ness, and to redefine their relationship. This time together was a blessing in the midst of tragedy. Mrs. M. felt more whole and integrated as a person during those last months than she had ever before in her life. As she peacefully went into a deep sleep, we all knew we had witnessed something special.

Her curve in the road was relatively easily managed. Unlike the Reverend, she did not have a near-death experience, but she remained intact mentally, spiritually, and emotionally. Her family simply had to adjust to an unpredictable turn of events that added a few more days to their time together. On the surface, there was no unfinished business or final revelation to explain her brief return to consciousness, but the few additional days they spent together were peaceful and easily tolerated.

Imagine a somewhat different scenario. Suppose the family had come together as described and Mrs. M. had gone into the deep sleep, but this time she awoke severely agitated, fearful, and confused. Medical understanding would attribute these symptoms to the metabolic changes associated with dehydration and her bodily systems shutting down. Mrs. M. and her family, however, would run the risk of having their wonderful coming together destroyed just before her death. How we respond to such crises says volumes about what it means to be a committed healer.

The personal disintegration that sometimes comes with such agitated delirium is profoundly disturbing, and requires a decisive response.[36] Because Mrs. M. was so close to death, doing blood tests to discern the cause(s) of the delirium would have been inappropriate. Our medical job here was primarily to relieve suffering, and to recapture the meaning and connectedness, if possible, the family had experienced over the past few months. This could probably be achieved only by sedating Mrs. M. to unconsciousness.[37] Her daughters would have to consent to the sedation on Mrs. M.'s behalf; they would also have to understand the importance of helping her escape this kind of terror, and accept the risk of hastening her inevitable death by a small amount of time. This risk would be more than counterbalanced by the inhumanity of continuing to let her suffer in this profound and dehumanizing way.

Physicians who commit to working with patients and families through the dying process must face unforeseeable turns in the patient's course. A commitment to face the unknown together, and to do everything in one's power to preserve and even enhance a patient's integrity and meaning, makes this one of medicine's richest, most rewarding, and at times most demanding endeavors. As these and other stories illustrate, the opportunities for growth and meaning are unsurpassed, yet the potential for disintegration is always lurking. To do this work, one must be both a romantic and a realist, both a guide and a student, and most of all, a committed partner.

References

1. *Concise Oxford English Dictionary*. (7th ed.) (1993). Oxford: Oxford University Press.
2. Smith RC, Hoppe RB. The patient's story: Integrating the patient- and physician-centered approaches to interviewing. *Ann Intern Med* 1991; 115:470–477.
3. Smith RC. *The Patient's Story. Integrated Patient-Doctor Interviewing*. Boston: Little, Brown and Company, 1996.
4. Pew-Fetzer Task Force on Advancing Psychosocial Health Education. (1994). *Health professions education and relationship-centered care: Report of the*

Pew-Fetzer Task Force on advancing psychosocial health education. San Francisco: Pew Health Professions Commission.
5. Peabody FW. The care of the patient. *N Engl J Med* 1927; 88:877–882.
6. Doyle D, Hanks GW, MacDonald N. *Oxford Textbook of Palliative Medicine*, 2nd ed. New York: Oxford University Press, 1998.
7. Quill TE, Dresser R, Brock DW. Rule of double effect: A critique of its role in end-of-life decision making. *N Engl J Med* 1997; 337:1768–1771.
8. Quinlan, In re, 137 N.J. Super. 227, 348 A. 2d 801 (Ch. Div., 1975), rev'd, 70 N.J. 10, 355 A. 2d 647, cert. denied sub nom. *Garger v. New Jersey*, 429 U.S. 922, 50 L. Ed. 2d 289, 97 S. Ct. 319 (1976) overruled in part, In re Conroy, 98 N.J. 321, 486 A. 2d 1209 (1985). 2000.
9. Carrillo JE, Green AR, Vetancourt JR. Cross-cultural primary care: A patient-based approach. *Ann Intern Med* 1999; 130:829–834.
10. Catanzaro A, Moser RJ. Health status of refugees from Vietnam, Laos, and Cambodia. *JAMA* 1982; 247:1303–1308.
11. Kleinman A, Eisenberg L, Good BJ. Culture, illness and cure. Clinical lessons from anthropologic and cross-cultural research. *Ann Intern Med* 1978; 88:251–258.
12. Bach PB, Craner LD, Warren JL, Begg CB. Racial differences in the treatment of early-stage lung cancer. *N Engl J Med* 1999; 341:1198–1205.
13. Schulman KA, Berlin JA, Harless W, Kerner JF, Sistrunk S, Gersh BJ, et al. The effect of race and sex on physicians' recommendations for cardiac catheterization. *N Engl J Med* 1999; 340:618–626.
14. Fairchild AL, Bayer R. Uses and abuses of Tuskegee. *Science* 1999; 284:919–921.
15. Duberstein PR, Conwell Y, Cox C, Podgorski CA, Glazer RS, Caine ED. Attitudes toward self-determined death: A survey of primary care physicians. *J Am Geriatr Soc* 1995; 43:395–400.
16. Dickinson GE, Tournier RE. A decade beyond medical school: A longitudinal study of physicians' attitudes toward death and terminally-ill patients. *Soc Sci Med* 1994; 38:1397–1400.
17. Neumann JK, Olive KE, McVeigh SD. Absolute versus relative values: effects of medical decisions and personality of patients and physicians. *South Med J* 1999; 92:871–876.
18. Hamilton DG. Believing in patients' beliefs: physician attunement to the spiritual dimension as a positive factor in patient healing and health. *Am J Hospice Palliat Care* 1998; 15:276–279.
19. Tversky A, Kahneman D. The framing of decisions and the psychology of choice. *Science* 1982; 211:453–458.
20. Quill TE, Brody H. Physician recommendations and patient autonomy: Finding a balance between physician power and patient choice. *Ann Intern Med* 1996; 125:763–769.
21. Bellett PS, Maloney MJ. The importance of empathy as an interviewing skill in medicine. *JAMA* 1991; 266:1831–1832.
22. Cohen-Cole SA. Interviewing the cardiac patient: I. A practical guide for assessing quality of life. *Qual Life Cardiovasc Care* 1985; (November/December):7–12.
23. Cohen-Cole SA, Bird J. Interviewing the cardiac patient: II. A practical guide for helping patients cope with their emotions. *Quality Life Cardiovasc Care* 1986; (January/February).
24. Byock I. *Dying Well: The Prospect for Growth at the End of Life*. New York: Riverhead Books, 1997.

25. Quill TE. Doctor, I want to die. Will you help me? *JAMA* 1993; 270:870–873.
26. Suchman AL, Matthews DA. What makes the patient–doctor relationship therapeutic? Exploring the connectional dimension of medical care. *Ann Intern Med* 1988; 108:125–130.
27. Karlawish JH, Quill TE, Meier DE. A consensus-based approach to providing palliative care to patients who lack decision-making capacity. ACP-ASIM End-of-Life Care Consensus Panel. *Ann Intern Med* 1999; 130:835–840.
28. Epstein RM. Mindful practice. *JAMA* 1999; 282(9):833–839.
29. Miller A. *Prisoners of Childhood. The Trauma of the Gifted Child and the Search for the True Self*. New York: Basic Books, 1981.
30. Novack DH, Epstein RM, Paulsen RH. Toward creating physician-healers: Fostering medical students' self-awareness, personal growth and well-being. *Acad Med* 1999; 74(5):516–520.
31. Wallston KA, Burger C, Smith RA, Baugher RJ. Comparing the quality of death for hospice and non-hospice cancer patients. *Med Care* 1988; 26:177–182.
32. Leplege A, Hunt S. The problem of quality of life in medicine. *JAMA* 1997; 278:47–50.
33. Cassell EJ. *The Nature of Suffering and the Goals of Medicine*. New York: Oxford University Press, 1991.
34. Frankl VE. *Man's Search for Meaning*. Boston: Beacon Press, 1959.
35. Quill TE. *A Midwife Through the Dying Process. Stories of Healing and Hard Choices at the End of Life*. Baltimore: Johns Hopkins University Press, 1996.
36. Casarect D, Inouye S. Diagnosis and Management of Delirium Near the End of Life. ACP-ASIM End-of-Life Care Consensus Panel. *Ann Intern Med* in press 2001.
37. Quill TE, Byock I. Responding to intractable terminal suffering: the role of terminal sedation and voluntary refusal of food and fluids. ACP-ASIM End-of-Life Care Consensus Panel. *Ann Intern Med* 2000; 132:408–414.

3

Death and Dignity: A Case of Individualized Decision Making

Diane was feeling tired and had a rash. A common scenario, although there was something subliminally worrisome about it that prompted me to check her blood count. Her hematocrit was 22, and her white-cell count was 4.3 with some metamyelocytes and unusual white cells. I wanted these results to be of viral origin, and I tried to deny what was staring me in the face. Perhaps in a repeated count they would disappear. I called Diane and relayed that her condition might be more serious than I had initially thought—that the blood test needed to be repeated and that if she felt worse, we might have to move quickly. When she pressed for the possibilities, I reluctantly opened the door to leukemia. Hearing the word seemed to make it exist. *"Oh, shit!"* she said. *"Don't tell me that."* Oh, shit! I thought. *I wish I didn't have to.*

Diane was no ordinary person (although no one I have ever come to know has been truly ordinary). She was raised in an alcoholic family and had felt alone for much of her life. She had vaginal cancer as a young woman. Through much of her adult life, she had struggled with depression and her own alcoholism. I had come to know, respect, and admire

This narrative was originally published in the *New England Journal of Medicine* 1991; 324:691–694.

her over the previous eight years as she confronted these problems and gradually overcame them. She was an incredibly clear, and at times brutally honest, thinker and communicator. As she took control of her life, she developed a strong sense of independence and confidence. In the previous three and a half years, her hard work had paid off. She was completely abstinent from alcohol, had established much deeper connections with her husband, college-age son, and several friends, and her business and her artistic work were blossoming. She felt she was really living fully for the first time.

Not surprisingly, the repeated blood count was abnormal, and a detailed examination of the peripheral blood smear showed myelocytes. I advised her to come into the hospital, explaining that we needed to do a bone marrow biopsy and make some decisions rapidly. She came to the hospital knowing what we would find. She was terrified, angry, and sad. Although we knew the odds, we both clung to the thread of possibility that it was something else.

The bone marrow evaluation confirmed the worst: acute myelomonocytic leukemia. In the face of this tragedy, we looked for signs of hope. This is an area of medicine in which technological intervention has been successful, with cures 25% of the time—long-term cures. As I probed the costs of these cures, I heard about induction chemotherapy (three weeks in the hospital, prolonged neutropenia, probable infectious complications, and hair loss; 75% of patients respond, 25% do not). For the survivors, this is followed by consolidation chemotherapy (with similar side effects; another 25% die, for a net survival of 50%). Those still alive, to have a reasonable chance of long-term survival, then need bone marrow transplantation (hospitalization for two months and whole-body irradiation, with complete killing of the bone marrow, infectious complications, and the possibility of graft-versus-host disease, with a survival of approximately 50%, or 25% of the original group). Though hematologists may argue over the exact percentages, they don't argue about the outcome of no treatment—certain death in days, weeks, or at most a few months.

Believing that delay was dangerous, our oncologist broke the news to Diane and made plans to insert a Hickman catheter and begin induction chemotherapy that afternoon. When I saw her shortly thereafter, she was enraged at his presumption that she would want treatment and devastated by the finality of the diagnosis. All she wanted to do was go home and be with her family. She had no further questions about treatment, and in fact had decided that she wanted none. Together we lamented her tragedy and the unfairness of life. Before she left, I felt the need to be sure that she and her husband understood that there was some risk in delay, that the problem was not going to go away, and that we needed to keep considering her options over the next several days. We agreed to meet in two days.

She returned in two days with her husband and son. They had talked extensively about her condition and options. She remained very clear about her wish not to undergo chemotherapy and to live whatever time she had left outside the hospital. As we explored her thinking further, it became clear that she was convinced she would die during the period of treatment and would suffer unspeakably in the process (from hospitalization, from lack of control over her body, from the side effects of chemotherapy, and from pain and anguish). Although I could offer support and my best effort to minimize her suffering if she chose treatment, there was no way I could say any of this would not occur. In fact, the last four patients with acute leukemia at our hospital had died very painful deaths in the hospital during various stages of treatment (a fact I did not share with her). Her family wished she would choose treatment but sadly accepted her decision. She articulated very clearly that it was she who would be experiencing all the side effects of treatment and that odds of 25% were not good enough for her to undergo so toxic a course of therapy, given her expectations of chemotherapy and hospitalization and the absence of a closely matched bone marrow donor. I had her state her understanding of the treatment, the odds, and what to expect if treatment was not pursued. I clarified a few misunderstandings, but she had a remarkable grasp of the options and implications.

I have been a longtime advocate of active, informed patient choice of treatment or nontreatment, and of a patient's right to die with as much control and dignity as possible. Yet there was something about her giving up a 25% chance of long-term survival in favor of almost certain death that disturbed me. I had seen Diane fight and use her considerable inner resources to overcome alcoholism and depression, and I half expected her to change her mind over the next week. Since the window of time in which effective treatment can be initiated is rather narrow, we met several times that week. We obtained a second hematology consultation and talked at length about the meaning and implications of treatment and nontreatment. She talked to a psychologist she had seen in the past. I gradually under-stood the decision from her perspective and became convinced that it was the right decision for her. We arranged for home hospice care (although at that time Diane felt reasonably well, was active, and looked healthy), left the door open for her to change her mind, and tried to anticipate how to keep her comfortable in the time she had left.

Just as I was adjusting to her decision, she broached another topic that would stretch me profoundly. It was important to Diane to maintain control of herself and her own dignity during the time remaining to her. When this was no longer possible, she clearly wanted to die. As a former director of a hospice program, I know how to use pain medicines to keep patients comfortable and lessen suffering. I explained the philosophy of comfort care, which I strongly believe in. Although Diane understood and appreciated this, she had known people who had lingered in what was called "relative comfort", and she wanted no part of it. When the time came, she wanted to take her life in the least painful way possible. Knowing of her desire for independence and her decision to stay in control, I thought this request made perfect sense. I acknowledged and explored this wish but also thought that it was out of the realm of accepted medical practice to assist her in this way, and that it was more than I could offer or promise. In our discussion, it became clear that preoccupation with her fear of a lingering death would interfere with Diane's getting the most out of the time she had left until she found a safe way to ensure her death. I feared the effects of a violent death on her family, the consequences of an ineffective suicide that would leave her lingering in precisely the state she dreaded so much, or the possibility that a family member would be forced to assist her, with all the legal and personal repercussions that would follow. She discussed this at length with her family. They believed that they should respect her choice. With this in mind, I told Diane that information was available from the Hemlock Society that might be helpful to her.

A week later, she phoned me with a request for barbiturates for sleep. Since I knew that this was an essential ingredient in a Hemlock Society suicide, I asked her to come to the office to talk things over. She was more than willing to protect me by participating in a superficial conversation about her insomnia, but it was important to me to know how she planned to use the drugs and to be sure that she was not in despair or overwhelmed in a way that might color her judgment. It was apparent from our discussion that she was having trouble sleeping, but it was also evident that the security of having enough barbiturates available to commit suicide when and if the time came would leave her secure enough to live fully and concentrate on the present. It was clear that she was not despondent and that in fact she was making deep, personal connections with her family and close friends. I made sure that she knew how to use the barbiturates for sleep, and also that she had researched the amount needed to commit suicide. We agreed to meet regularly, and she promised to meet with me before taking her life, to ensure that all other avenues had been exhausted. I wrote the prescription with an uneasy feeling about the boundaries I was exploring— spiritual, legal, professional, and personal. Yet I also felt strongly that I was setting her free to get the most out of the time she had left, and to maintain dignity and control on her own terms until her death.

The next several months were very intense and important for Diane. Her son stayed home from college, and they were able to be with one another and say much that had not been said earlier. Her husband did his work at home so that he and Diane could spend more time together. She spent time with her closest friends. I had her come into the hospital for a conference with our residents, at which she illustrated in a most profound and personal way the importance of informed decision making, the right to refuse treatment, and the extraordinarily personal impact of her illness and her interaction with the medical system. There were emotional and physical hardships as well. She had periods of intense sadness and anger. Several times she became very weak, but she received transfusions as an outpatient and responded with a marked improvement of symptoms. She had two serious infections that responded surprisingly well to empirical courses of oral antibiotics. After three tumultuous months, there were two weeks of relative calm and well-being, and fantasies of a miracle began to surface.

Unfortunately, we had no miracle. Bone pain, weakness, fatigue, and fevers began to dominate her life. Although the hospice workers, family members, and I tried our best to minimize her suffering and promote comfort, it was clear that the end was approaching. Diane's immediate future held what she feared the most—increasing discomfort, dependence, and hard choices between pain and sedation. She called up her closest friends and asked them to come over to say good-bye, telling them that she would be leaving soon. As we had agreed, she let me know as well. When we met, it was clear that she knew what she was doing, that she was sad and frightened to be leaving, but that she would be even more terrified to stay and suffer. In our tearful good-bye, she promised a reunion in the future at her favorite spot on the edge of Lake Geneva, with dragons swimming in the sunset.

Two days later, her husband called to say that Diane had died. She had said her final good-byes to her husband and son that morning, and asked them to leave her alone for an hour. After an hour, which must have seemed an eternity, they found her on the couch lying very still and covered by her favorite shawl. There was no sign of struggle. She seemed to be at peace. They called me for advice about how to proceed. When I arrived at their house, Diane indeed seemed peaceful. Her husband and son were quiet. We talked about what a remarkable person she had been. They seemed to have no doubts about the course she had chosen or about their coopera- tion, although the unfairness of her illness and the finality of her death were overwhelming to us all.

I called the medical examiner to inform him that a hospice patient had died. When asked about the cause of death, I said, "Acute leukemia." He said that was fine and that we should call a funeral director. Although acute leukemia was the truth, it was not the whole story. Yet any mention of suicide would have given rise to a police investigation and probably brought the arrival of an ambulance crew for resuscitation. Diane would have become a "coroner's case," and the decision to perform an autopsy would have been made at the discretion of the medical examiner. The family or I could have been subject to criminal prosecution, and I to professional review, for our roles in support of Diane's choices. Although I truly believe that the family and I gave her the best care possible, allowing her to define her limits and directions as much as possible, I am not sure the law, society, or the medical profession would agree. So I said "Acute leukemia" to protect all of us, to protect Diane from an invasion into her past and her body, and to continue to shield society from the knowledge of the degree of suffering that people often undergo in the process of dying. Suffering can be lessened to some extent, but in no way eliminated or made benign, by the careful intervention of a competent, caring physician, given current social constraints.

Diane taught me about the range of help I can provide if I know people well and if I allow them to say what they really want. She taught me about life, death, and honesty, and about taking charge and facing tragedy squarely when it strikes. She taught me that I can take small risks for people I really know and care about. Although I did not assist in her suicide directly, I helped indirectly to make it possible, successful, and relatively painless. Although I know we have measures to help control pain and lessen suffering, to think that people do not suffer in the process of dying is an illusion. Prolonged dying can occasionally be peaceful, but more often the role of the physician and family is limited to lessening but not eliminating severe suffering.

I wonder how many families and physicians secretly help patients over the edge into death in the face of such severe suffering. I wonder how many severely ill or dying patients secretly take their lives, dying alone in despair. I wonder if the image of Diane's final aloneness will persist in the minds of her family, or if they will remember more the intense, meaningful months they had together before she died. I wonder whether Diane struggled in that last hour, and whether the Hemlock Society's way of death by suicide is the most benign. I wonder why Diane, who gave so much to so many of us, had to be alone for the last hour of her life. I wonder whether I will see Diane again, on the shore of Lake Geneva at sunset, with dragons swimming on the horizon.

4

Partnerships in the Care of the Dying

Patients approaching the end of their lives face frightening uncertainties and unanswered questions. As the dying process unfolds, will they experience pain that is hard to control? Will their integrity as persons stay intact? Will they remain in control of their bodies, minds, and spirits? As patients and their families try to imagine the future, they may wonder about their medical practitioners. Are they professionals who can be counted on to remain responsive no matter what happens? Do they have expertise in this phase of life? Are they going to listen and keep the patient's values in the foreground? Can they be counted on as friends as well as professionals?

Medical partnerships have special meaning at this point in the patient–physician relationship. The answers to these questions about commitment, responsiveness, and keeping the patient's values in the foreground should be answered resoundingly in the affirmative. Although medical partners cannot guarantee an easy road, or even a course that will not include severe suffering or threats to bodily or psychic integrity, they can promise to remain connected and help the patient face whatever future challenges might present themselves.

A partner is defined as someone who shares in a common action or endeavor with another.[1] In law or business, partners formally associate with each other in joint ventures, usually sharing similar risks and profits. In medicine, however, the risks and benefits of partnership are different for patients, family members, and health care providers. For terminally ill patients, the potential benefits of partnership with a skilled medical practitioner are clear. Current and future suffering can be addressed regardless of whether it is biological (pain and other physical symptoms), psychological (anxiety, fear, depression), social (family problems, financial issues), or spiritual (meaning of this life, reconciliation, forgiveness) in nature. Such a complex, multidimensional process cannot be the province of just one person such as a physician, but the medical partner can help access professionals from multiple disciplines, as needed, to assist the patient and family contend with what emerges as most important.

Although it is easy to see how severely ill patients and their families benefit from having medical partners, the gains for medical professionals are sometimes less immediately tangible. On the surface, most professionals who are not working on a volunteer basis get paid for their involvement. For physicians, however, the level of reimbursement for end-of-life care is a fraction of what can be earned by providing more technologically driven care. Furthermore, in acute care settings, insurance reimbursement flows to multiple providers and to the institution itself as long as aggressive treatment continues, and it dries to a trickle as soon as there is a shift to a more palliative approach. Why, then, do physicians and other medical professionals become involved in end-of-life care?

Most physicians go into the medical profession to serve patients, with the hope of curing or perhaps of staving off death, but also with a desire to relieve suffering and to be connected in a meaningful way with their patients. Patients want to be treated with caring and respect by medical practitioners, whose expertise and honesty can help them make the best decisions possible even when disease cannot be cured and death cannot be postponed. Physicians who engage in these intimate partnerships with their dying patients clearly gain as much as they give, but the gains are probably more personal and existential than financial. For many physicians, caring for patients at the end of life helps them reconnect with the values that originally drove them toward the practice of medicine, or perhaps helps them identify these values for the first time.

Critical Elements of the Medical Partnership

Five critical elements of the medical partnership are explored below and summarized in Table 4–1.

Sharing Power and Expertise

As medical professionals and patients, often with their families, come together to form partnerships, they may or may not have a history of working together.

TABLE   4–1. Five   Critical   Elements   of   Medical
Partnerships

Sharing power and expertise

Mutually influencing and understanding one another

Clarifying commonness and differences

Negotiating differences

Ultimately patient-centered

In either case, they must establish a way of working together that allows the sharing of power and expertise.

Patients have a wealth of personal experience, both medical and otherwise, that might be brought to bear on medical decisions. Furthermore, they may have very personal values about autonomy, control, dependence, and/or the meaning of various types of diseases or interventions. One patient with an incurable cancer might view a transition to hospice as an unacceptable form of "giving up," and want to pursue experimental therapy despite its invasiveness and its low probability of success. Another patient, identically situated, might view experimental therapy as meaningless, welcoming instead the promise of hospice in improving quality of life for the time that remains. For the decision-making process to be truly informed and personalized, each patient's personal experience has to be integrated into it.

However, medical decisions cannot be driven exclusively by patients' limited medical experiences. Decision making must also be based on input from knowledgeable, experienced medical professionals. Physicians should use their medical expertise, their ability to research the medical literature, and their access to other professionals with specialized skills to help patients and families understand medicine's capabilities and limitations. The patient's physician-as-partner has a responsibility to integrate this information and look at it in the context of his or her own personal and professional experience, as well as to incorporate the values and experience of the patient. This knowledge and experience should form the basis of an open and honest conversation with the patient and family about realistic options, including any recom-mendations that the physician may have about the best treatment course.[2] Physicians also have a responsibility to control proper access to medical interventions ranging from opioids for proper pain management to invasive experimental therapy.

What did Diane and I bring to our partnership from the outset of her final illness? We had worked together for eight years, including times of intense confrontation when I was trying to help her overcome her problems with alcoholism and depression. In the eight years before she was diagnosed with leukemia, she had been living her life more fully and with more joy than ever before. At first glance, one might think that such experience would make her willing to risk substantial suffering in the interests of sustaining life. Yet Diane also strongly valued her physical integrity. She was fearful of having her body invaded by potentially toxic medications or placed in the hands of strangers. Diane's struggles with prior illnesses, including vaginal cancer, had left her unwilling to accept further suffering unless she was assured a successful outcome after taking the medication.

I, on the other hand, brought to the partnership a strong belief in the power of medical technology to prolong life and at times even cure disease, but I also had substantial clinical experience where invasive treatment had been continued far beyond its usefulness. I brought faith in hospice care to provide an important alternative to technology-dominated approaches to the end of life. I am willing to talk openly with patients and families when I feel that their level of suffering is high and their prognosis is poor enough to make a transition. Diane's illness had a 25% chance of cure, a reasonably good prognosis in my eyes. In spite of Diane's reservations, I initially felt she should try invasive treatment, and strongly recommended that course to her. I did, however, believe that it was ultimately her decision, since (as Diane would repeatedly remind me!) it was she and not I who would be going through the treatment process. This particular treatment, a combination of chemotherapy, radiation, and bone marrow transplantation, was not something to be undertaken lightly. Thus, I offered to Diane medical expertise, a deep caring about her well-being, a willingness to challenge her if I thought she was making a bad decision, but also a belief that she should be the final decision maker about medical matters that affected her body and person.

Mutual Influence and Understanding

There is nothing passive about a healthy partnership. Overly simplistic notions of autonomy suggest that to protect a patient's integrity and decision-making authority, the physician should present information, options, and statistically relevant risks and benefits, then follow through with a patient's decision.[2] Physician paternalism has been equated with controlling and dominating the patient, subjugating him or her to a passive role. Whereas it has the potential to overpower the patient, paternalism also has some positive elements, such as using one's expertise and experience to do what seems best for the patient. Paternalistic physicians genuinely care about what happens to their patients, and want to use their knowledge and skill on the patient's behalf. An overzealous, controlling physician may want the patient to follow his or her direction in all circumstances, yet it is also possible for physicians to become too passive in their efforts to protect patient autonomy.

The counterbalancing force that will protect patients from being unduly influenced is the capacity to listen to and learn from the patient's experience. When patient and physician clearly agree on a course, this formal process of mutual exploration and influence may be less essential. However, when there is a difference of opinion about how to proceed, or when the clinical options are unclear or controversial, the need for an open and honest sharing of ideas and concerns is compelling. Through this exchange, each party's views and positions can be fully explored, so a deeper understanding can be reached that better reflects the patient's unique values and clinical situation. Such mutual exchanges also respect patient autonomy in a way that providing information and then simply following the patient's initial choice does not.[2] Later in this chapter, I will describe how Diane and I influenced each other at three critical points in the course of her terminal illness. Her choices, and the meaning we each attached to them, evolved as a result of that process of mutual influence.

Clarification of Commonness and Differences

Whenever there is disagreement or uncertainty about how to proceed with clinical decision making, it is useful to try to fully understand where there is agreement and disagreement. Not infrequently, disagreement about a method of treatment may reflect a difference in understanding about the goals of treatment or the nature of the problem. This is particularly true at the end of life, where the goals of treatment may need to be scaled back and the extent of the problem may be difficult to fully grasp. Before trying to resolve a conflict, it is useful to step back and make sure the areas of agreement and disagreement are fully understood. Sometimes this shifts the level of the conversation to a more critical dimension that underlies the perceived conflict. This approach has been adapted from the work of Aaron Lazare, who developed it for use within a psychiatric walk-in clinic. It has wide applicability to clinical medicine.[3] Table 4–2 summarizes some of the dimensions of conflict that have relevance to end-of-life care.

Diagnosis and prognosis

In end-of-life care, diagnosis is usually not in question, especially in the United States, where truth telling is a standard of care. There will be exceptional circumstances where a diagnosis is withheld from a particular patient for cultural reasons (for some Russian-Jewish immigrants, cancer is equated with a death sentence and it is deemed cruel to tell the patient), but for the most part patients know their diagnosis even when they are being protected.[4-6] On the other hand, many patients do not know or understand the seriousness of the diagnosis or its actual prognosis. The patient, family members, or health

TABLE 4–2. Clarifying Commonness and Differences:
Potential Dimensions of Conflict

Diagnosis and prognosis

Goals of treatment

Methods of treatment

Conditions of treatment

Relationship

Psychological and emotional factors

Spirituality and religion

care providers may have unrealistically optimistic or pessimistic views of the patient's prognosis that will then drive future decisions. Furthermore, information about prognosis is inherently uncertain and probabilistic, and therefore it is difficult to interpret in light of a particular patient. Patients with severe congestive heart failure, for example, may have a 50% chance of dying in six months but a 25% chance of living two years or more.[7] Diane's initial diagnosis of acute myelomonocytic leukemia meant she had a 25% chance of cure with aggressive chemotherapy, radiation, and bone marrow transplantation, yet the converse was that she had a 75% chance of dying during the course of a very demanding treatment. Part of the challenge of this dimension is to have the patient, family, and physician achieve a common understanding about diagnosis and prognosis, including its inherent complexity when applied to a particular patient.

Goals of treatment

The two main goals of medical treatment are to prolong life and to alleviate human suffering.[8] Many times in the course of treatment, these goals are in conflict. For example, in the treatment of acute leukemia, we ask patients to endure aggressive chemotherapy, radiation, and bone marrow transplantation, each associated with iatrogenic suffering, in the interest of prolonging their lives. Most of those who are lucky enough to survive look back and say that the suffering was worth it, though they also say the treatment was much more invasive and difficult than they had envisioned. Family members of those who do not survive may question the wisdom of their original decision, and say if they had a crystal ball and had known the outcome, they would never have allowed their loved one to endure such suffering before death. As a patient's prognosis gets poorer and poorer, and as quality of life diminishes and suffering increases, the goals of treatment may change. In many circumstances, palliative treatments (opioids for pain) can be provided in parallel with life-prolonging treatments (chemotherapy attacking cancer cells). Nevertheless, as death

approaches, relief of suffering usually takes precedence, even at the risk of indirectly shortening life, as with the use of very high doses of opioids to treat accelerating pain or shortness of breath toward the very end.[9] (In fact, apart from
these exceptional circumstances, pain management usually lengthens life rather
than shortens it, and certainly contributes to the patient's quality of life.)

Methods of treatment

Treatment methods are dictated in part by what is medically available and
of proven benefit, but also by the patient's goals given the diagnosis and prognosis. For example, one patient I recently encountered with widely metastatic
bladder cancer had failed all treatments of proven benefit. He appeared to be
suffering severely from disfiguring, painful bony lesions, and in my mind was
an excellent candidate for hospice care. Our goal, I thought, should be to maximize his quality of life for the time that remained without adding to his suffering. To my surprise, he found no hope or meaning in the promise of hospice,
and wanted instead to treat his disease with experimental chemotherapy, even
if it was unlikely to work and very likely to make him feel more sick for his final
days. His goal was to fight his disease to his last breath, using any means possible, even if it worsened his quality of life. He was willing to accept many
standard palliative treatments, including around-the-clock high-dose opioids
for pain and steroids for brain swelling. After extensive discussions, he also
accepted a do-not-resuscitate order, since he understood that cardiopulmonary
resuscitation would not help him if his condition deteriorated to that point.
Disagreements about methods often reflect a lack of agreement on other issues,
and it is generally useful to explore these other issues before negotiating
about methods. In this case, once I understood the patient's goals and his
willingness to accept the increased suffering that came with experimental
treatment, we were able to agree on methods that combined aggressive and
palliative treatments.

Conditions of treatment

Conditions can be placed on further treatment by either the physician or
the patient. For example, a patient with renal failure who is prepared to die
and is contemplating stopping dialysis treatments might be asked to undergo
a psychiatric evaluation or a trial of antidepressant therapy before making a
final decision. The physician, in turn, could make a commitment to support
this patient's request once treatable depression or other factors that might
be clouding judgment are excluded. When Diane was considering forgoing
potentially life-sustaining aggressive treatment of her leukemia, I insisted
that she explore the issues with a second consulting hematologist, as well as
with her former psychotherapist. Conditions of treatment may go both ways.
Upon entering a hospice program, a patient might place any of the following

conditions on the continuation of a doctor–patient relationship: a willingness to prescribe pain medications, to do home visits, or to be responsive to extremes of any future suffering. This information is of particular importance if patients or families have witnessed difficult deaths with unresponsive physicians in the past.

Relationship

When a doctor and patient have a long-standing relationship, especially one that has weathered prolonged illness, they may have a strong base of shared experience going into the patient's final illness. However, many seriously ill patients do not have this luxury. They may not have needed much medical care in the past, or they have changed doctors due to the nature of modern health plans, or they live in an area where they are unfamiliar with the medical community, or they have been unable to afford even basic medical care. In all of these circumstances, defining the nature of the medical relationship and the extent of the partnership is essential.

Diane and I were fortunate to have a long-standing relationship in which we had worked through serious challenges with her alcoholism and depression. We were able to be honest and direct with each other. Diane, in particular, had an ability to cut to the core of issues and ask difficult questions. She had confidence that I would try to answer these questions to the best of my ability, and that I was not frightened by her forthrightness or her need to stay in control. This foundation made the difficult decision making that we had to pursue a little easier. If we had not had this shared history, then our initial interaction and negotiation would have been a testing ground for our relationship, and for the type of partnership that was possible. The type of relationship that each party is looking for can sometimes be articulated and negotiated in advance when the doctor and patient are strangers, but for patients to ultimately trust in the relationship, the carrying through of agreed-upon commitments must always be demonstrated over time.

Psychological and emotional factors

When patients are on the verge of an ethically and clinically challenging decision, such as choosing experimental therapy, stopping a life support, or considering a physician-assisted death, the possibility that their judgment is being distorted by depression, anxiety, an organic brain process, or external psychosocial factors must be considered.[10] When patients are aware and accepting of this possibility, they may welcome a psychological evaluation to make sure they are making the best decision possible. More commonly, however, patients may feel they have a clear notion of what they need, and may resent the notion that others believe their thinking might be less than clear. Furthermore, an evaluation of depression can be challenging in these circumstances, since many of the symptoms of severe illness (fatigue, sleep disturbance, sadness, preoccupation with death and dying) mimic those of depression.[11] It is important not to "over-normalize" (anyone would be depressed under these circumstances) or "over-pathologize" (he must be depressed if he is talking about stopping life supports). Skilled mental health professionals can be invaluable in sorting out these issues. It helps if such practitioners have experience treating severely medically ill patients.

Spirituality and religion

When a doctor and patient have similar views of religion or spirituality, this may help to cement their partnership. On the other hand, physicians as a group tend to be nonreligious compared to the population at large,[12-17] while patients who are faced with severe illness often embrace a spiritual path in order to make sense of what has happened to them. The physician, or some member of the health care team, should take responsibility for exploring spiritual issues with the patient.[18] If a patient is part of a religious community, then perhaps his or her own clergy can become involved. If not, the responsibility might fall to the hospital or hospice chaplain. Medical practitioners and patients may have very different views about why people get sick, why some recover and others do not, and what role, if any, religion and spirituality play in the healing process. Although Diane felt it was unfair that she became so ill, she did not see her illness as any form of punishment, nor was she angry at God for what happened. She did not participate in organized religion as an adult, and she was not interested in reconnecting with the religion of her childhood. She did have a strong vision of an afterlife, where she felt she would be going, and she believed that extremes of suffering during the dying process served no meaningful spiritual or existential purpose for her. Since her views in this regard were very close to mine, they tended to solidify and deepen our relationship as we faced her unknown future together.

Negotiation of Differences

Similar negotiation strategies are used in business, law, diplomacy, and medicine. A simple yet effective strategy for negotiation has been developed by Fisher and Ury based on their observations of skilled negotiators in a variety of fields.[19] It is outlined in Table 4–3. I will briefly describe some of these strategies, then illustrate them in the next section, showing how Diane and I negotiated at several difficult points in her terminal course.

A common negotiation flaw that affects even skilled negotiators is to engage in power struggles with the potential partner. Here, a search for common ground is overshadowed by determining who is right and who is wrong about

TABLE 4–3. Negotiation of Differences

Listen and learn about each other's position
Separate the person from the problem
Invent solutions of mutual gain
Call in a third party
Take a "time-out"
Give in on nonessential areas
Explore the likely effects of each choice
Know your bottom line

a particular issue. A need to win takes over, and a potential partner has now become an adversary. In medicine, such power struggles are fraught with hazard, since the patient, made vulnerable by disease, may not be able to stand up to the physician, who may think he or she knows the best course for the patient. Many otherwise independent, highly capable patients follow their doctor's directives against their own better judgment simply because standing up to a physician is too threatening. Perhaps the most common example of this is when a highly trained subspecialist recommends another round of invasive experimental therapy, and the patient accepts simply out of fear of losing the physician.

The first step out of such power struggles is to "separate the person from the problem," which means to disengage from the personal battle of wills and redirect the discussion to try to achieve a common understanding of the patient's problem and the nature of the disagreement. Each party must listen thoroughly to the other's position with an open mind, and without arguing or interrupting. These negotiations frequently also include family members if they are intimately involved in the patient's care plan or decision-making processes. Once all parties have been thoroughly heard, clarifying commonness and differences along the dimensions of conflict outlined in Table 4–2 is important. Most commonly, a disagreement about treatment methods actually reflects differences in understanding about prognosis or goals of treatment. Defining the dimensions where there is agreement helps reinforce the bonds that unite the partnership and puts the disagreement in perspective. Sometimes disagreement at one level disappears once differences in understanding at other levels are clarified. As one works on an area of disagreement, all efforts should be made to find new solutions where both parties can win. For example, the patient might agree to a time-limited trial of chemotherapy to see how it is tolerated and if it appears to show any immediate response. The physician might agree to simultaneously provide more aggressive palliation of symptoms, including regular use of around-the-clock opioids and spiritual counseling around end-of-life issues.

When an impasse remains after good-faith negotiation, taking a "time-out" so that both parties can consider their positions away from each other can be useful. There are a few instances, such as a patient with acute myocardial infarction, where minutes of delay can make a big difference in outcome. More commonly, such as when a patient decides to proceed with experimental chemotherapy for advanced cancer, the probability of success is not changed with delays of days or even a few weeks. In Diane's case, such a delay allowed time for her to reconsider her decision and to seek opinions from other professionals and laypersons whose counsel she trusted. As the emotional shock of the decision wore off, I genuinely thought (and hoped) Diane would change her mind. The probability of success with treatment was not significantly changed by the two-week hiatus. It gave her the opportunity to fully explore her decision and its consequences. I tried to persuade her to try treatment, promising that she could stop at any time if her suffering became unacceptably harsh, but she remained steadfast in her belief that she would be one of the 75% who did not survive. If she had agreed, she would most likely have spent her last months in the hospital being invaded by treatment rather than at home with her family.

As we explored the likely consequences of each other's position, virtually every consultant wanted to be certain that Diane understood that death was a certainty without treatment, and that death from leukemia—probably from bleeding or overwhelming infection—was likely to be difficult. Having educated herself about the predictable side effects of chemotherapy, whole-body radiation, and bone marrow transplantation, Diane would counter that such invasive processes were even less desirable in her eyes. Diane's bottom line was that it would be she, not us, who would experience the burdens of either course so it was her decision to make. Diane and I were in agreement that this momentous choice between a series of bad options was hers, and I would support her no matter what the future held.

Ultimately Patient-Centered

The patient is the one with the disease, and the one who most fundamentally gains the benefits and bears the burdens of treatment decisions. The patient's family, broadly defined as others with a close, caring relationship with the patient, also have interests and need to make sense of the patient's decisions. However, their interests are slightly less central, since it is not their own body and soul that hang in the balance. The physician's primary interest should be doing what is best for patients—caring for and about patients as if they were members of the physician's own immediate family. Conflict between a physician and patient can be about power and control, but it can also be about a genuine difference in opinion about what is best for the patient. Thus, even though medical decisions are ultimately patients' to make because patients have final authority over their own bodies, this process of negotiation about the best course is in patients' best interests. In a healthy medical partnership, both parties care deeply about what happens to the patient. This intense effort to influence each other reflects better respect for patient autonomy than would simply providing information and then passively following the patient's lead or wishes.

Even though the patient has the final word, this does not mean that physicians should violate fundamental values in the interest of patient autonomy. Although there were several challenging points in Diane's terminal course, the most ethically controversial moment was my responding to her request for barbiturates to sleep, which I knew she would be stockpiling in case she needed them in the future. I was sure that Diane was not depressed and that the request was consistent with her long-standing personal values. Yet I also had to ask myself if I could live with myself ethically and spiritually if I provided the prescription and she subsequently took it. Furthermore, I had to ask myself if I was willing to face the professional and legal consequences of her act should it be discovered.

I finally decided that our partnership and friendship was strong enough for me to take these risks on her behalf, and that I could live with the consequences of my participation. If I were not willing to provide the prescription because of moral, legal, or clinical reservations, I should then try to stretch myself to decide what I could promise in the hope of lessening her fears. For example, would I be willing to provide terminal sedation if her suffering became extreme? If so, would this be acceptable to Diane? Although I believe physicians should not participate in acts that are outside their moral framework, I also believe they should use the process of negotiation to try to find common ground, and to invent potential solutions that are acceptable to patients and themselves.

Partnership in Action: Three Critical Decisions in the Case of Diane

My partnership with Diane and her family was already well-formed when Diane was diagnosed with leukemia. Because of this, there was never a significant question about the nature of our relationship or my commitment to see the process through no matter what the future held or what decisions were made. Nevertheless, there were three points in her terminal course where we had to work hard to define common ground using the clarification and negotiation skills outlined above.

Deciding Whether to Pursue Aggressive Therapy

Diane's leukemia had about a 25% chance for cure at the time of diagnosis. Because we regularly treat diseases with much poorer odds, the physicians and other medical personnel involved in Diane's case assumed she would want to begin treatment immediately. The staff had a recollection of the last four patients we had treated aggressively, all of whom had died difficult deaths in the hospital during various stages of treatment, and they irrationally believed that this improved Diane's statistical odds of a good response. Even when she initially refused treatment, I believed she would change her mind when given a chance to think things over. Although our original disagreement was at the level of methods of treatment, it became clear after further negotiation that it reflected a difference in opinion about prognosis and goals. To Diane, a 25% chance of survival was very poor odds, and she began asking hard questions about what happened to the other 75%. She learned that approximately one-third died in each of the three phases of treatment: chemotherapy, whole-body radiation therapy, and bone marrow transplantation. Diane did not have a bone marrow donor with a close genetic match, so her odds may have been even poorer. She fully informed herself about the side effects of treatment, which were likely to occur whether she lived or died in the course of treatment. Since Diane strongly believed that she would be among the 75% who do not survive, subjecting herself to additional suffering made no sense to her. She therefore wanted to devote all of her energy to minimizing suffering and making the most of the time she had left.

One of the more challenging areas to consider in our negotiation was the potential role of depression in her decision-making process. Diane had a history of depression and substance abuse, and had suffered from vaginal cancer earlier in her life. She had overcome these problems, but her losses and history might well have confounded her perception of this decision. On the other hand, Diane had shown great strength overcoming these problems, and had been leading a full, enjoyable life with excellent family connections at the time of her diagnosis. Diane was strong-willed and wanted to be in control of her life. She lamented the unfairness of the diagnosis coming at this stage in her life, and she resented the oncologist's assuming she would want to begin treatment the next day. Before we took the "time-out" to let her go home to think things over, I asked her to seek a second opinion from another hematologist who had a very gentle, collaborative style. I also requested that she see her psychologist of many years to make sure she was covering all bases. Diane was sure she was thinking clearly and was not depressed, but she agreed to see her therapist because of the momentous nature of her decision. Diane's therapist found her to be cognitively clear and not clinically depressed, and offered to meet with her at any time she desired in the future. As she became more informed about what was required in aggressive treatment, Diane became even more resolute that she wanted no part of it. If her time was limited, she would spend as much of it as possible at home with her family.

I also involved her family at all stages in the decision making. I had hoped at first that they might convince her to undertake treatment. Although her son and husband both wanted her to seriously consider aggressive treatment, they, too, believed that this was her decision to make. They helped by attending all of her appointments with her, asking hard questions of all of the consultants, and being an extra set of eyes and ears. Without question, we all had Diane's best interests at heart, and none of us liked any of her options.

We tried to invent new solutions. What about trying treatment to see if it was tolerable to her? She could stop at any time if the going got too hard. Diane rejected this option; she felt that the severity of the particular chemotherapy regimen she would need was too invasive to even try. We then explored hospice care, where all interventions would be devoted to improving and sustaining her quality of life. A hospice approach was clearly what Diane wanted. Her son would take time off from school, and her husband would work from home. Access to palliative care providers from a number of disciplines (nursing, social work, clergy, volunteers, and home health aides) would be provided. Although the plan made sense given my understanding of Diane's point of view, I left open the possibility of her changing her mind at any time and shifting her focus toward cure. However, after our extensive exploration and negotiation, I now doubted that such a change in goals and treatment would occur.

The Possibility of an Escape in the Future

Diane welcomed the promise of hospice. We would devote all of our energies to maintaining her quality of life and relieving her suffering. Pain and other physical symptoms would be managed aggressively, and she would spend the majority of her energy achieving closure with her family and working on her art. Once again, Diane asked difficult questions. The opening of this dialogue began with a query about methods, as she asked if she could be given some barbiturates for sleep. Based on our prior conversations, it was clear to me that she was seeking a potential escape if her suffering became unacceptable in the future. She had seen friends suffer before dying in hospice programs, and she was particularly fearful of dying in severe pain or out of control of her mind or body. Diane had carefully explored the prognosis of untreated leukemia, and had learned that patients frequently die of uncontrolled bleeding or from overwhelming infection. She asked about what dying of these complications might be like. If that happened in her future, her goal would change to ending her life as a way to escape such extreme suffering. Furthermore, she would worry about an unacceptable end until she had developed a plan that she could count on.

The roles of emotion and spirituality needed to be explored as well. Was this an unrealistic and pathological need to control her future, or was there a reality base to her fears? Was this a form of suicide, or was it more an effort at self-preservation? Diane was a very independent, proud woman whose body had been invaded medically once before when she had vaginal cancer. Her memories of this process were painful on many levels, and she had no desire to revisit them. Furthermore, her clarity of mind was one of her most defining personal characteristics. When that was gone, continued life would have no meaning for her. It did not make any sense to her to devote her last months to connecting with her family, only to die in a way that for her would be undignified and humiliating. After talking with her and her family, as well as others involved in her care, I know that Diane was clearly acting in a way that was consistent with her long-standing values and beliefs. For Diane, ending her life in this way would be an act of self-preservation and not self-destruction.

Diane and I had agreement about her goals and about the nature of the problem. Our negotiation occurred now at the level of methods. I reiterated that I would not withhold pain medication, even if the amount she required could hasten her death.[9,20] Although she appreciated this, she was more concerned about mental confusion, extreme physical dependence, hemorrhaging, and overwhelming infection than she was about pain. We talked about the possibility of terminal sedation under such circumstances.[10] She found this option to be unacceptable, since mental alertness was a core element of her being, and dying sedated in an iatrogenic coma seemed worse than death to her. She also feared that the lasting images her family would carry of her in such a condition might undermine the high-quality experience they were sharing now.

This led us to my prescribing barbiturates that would have a double purpose—they could be used as a sleeping medication, or, if taken all at once, to end life. Diane felt that having the medication in hand would reassure her of a possible escape, and that she could then focus her energies on matters of life closure.[21] I agreed to provide a prescription subject to two conditions. First, she would have to get information about dosing from the Hemlock Society, which at the time was the only source for such material. I did not have access to such information, and I also felt she should take as much responsibility in the process as possible. Second, she would agree to meet with me face-to-face before taking the medication so that I could be sure that every alternative had been exhausted and that she was thinking and seeing her situation clearly. Diane agreed to both conditions, and I subsequently provided the prescriptions.

Outside of Oregon, providing this kind of assistance is illegal, although it is not vigorously prosecuted by law enforcement provided it remains outside the attention of the media. In Chapters 9 and 12, I explore in more detail how to evaluate and respond to such requests in this uncertain legal environment. One of the consequences of this passive prohibition is that these profound decisions are made in secret. I would have appreciated second opinions from palliative care specialists, ethicists, and/or psychiatrists; I usually solicit second opinions for other potentially life-ending decisions, such as stopping life support. I was fortunate to have trusted colleagues, some of whom had faced similar dilemmas in the past, whom I could confidentially consult about Diane's case. I also talked with several hospice nurses involved in Diane's care about her mental state. They each commented that working with a patient like Diane who was forthright in her opinions and faced death so openly was what had attracted them to hospice work in the first place. Despite these opinions, I knew that a more formal consultative process would have been better and safer for Diane.

Diane's Decision to End Life

Diane lived for three months after enrolling in the hospice program. She had healing contact with her family, said good-bye to the people she loved, and gradually prepared for her death. She wanted to live as long as her life had quality and meaning (by her definition), and she took several life-prolonging treatments, including transfusions and antibiotics, in hopes of gaining some additional time. The hospice team members loved to visit her, in part because of her candor and clear thinking, but also because she appeared to be making the most of her limited time with respect to family healing. She kept the barbiturates I had prescribed in a safe place; it provided the security she needed to spend her energy on more important matters. Her pain was easily controlled with regular use of opioids, and her first few infections responded surprisingly well to potent oral antibiotics that she could take at home.

Unfortunately, but entirely predictably, her condition abruptly began to deteriorate after an initial three-month period during which she felt surprisingly well. Her pain from extensive bone involvement now required increasing doses of opioids, to the point where she had to make trade-offs between the mental clarity that was so important to her and pain relief. She then developed shaking chills and high fevers that did not respond to antibiotics. With her severely compromised immune system, her life expectancy was now days to at most a week or two, no matter what our approach. That time would have been Diane's worst nightmare—increased physical dependence, decreased mental clarity, and trade-offs between pain and sedation. She was dying, and she understood and accepted it. She had promised to meet with me face-to-face before taking her overdose, and she fulfilled this condition of our agreement.

We reviewed the various levels of our understanding to make sure that no stone had been left unturned. This was too important a decision not to double-check each dimension. Diane's goals were still to relieve suffering and in particular to avoid extremes of suffering at the end; for her this meant relief not only from pain and other physical symptoms, but also from mental clouding and physical dependency. Since her death was inevitable at this stage, these goals made sense to me as well. Her problem and its prognosis were clearly understood. She was dying of leukemia, and she had already lived longer and had a better quality of life for that time than we had expected. We also knew the likely sequence of events caused by overwhelming infection, which included high fever, low blood pressure, severe chills, a gradual loss of consciousness, and eventual death. We checked for the potential confounding effects of emotion: She clearly understood her situation and options. She was sad, but not depressed. She did not want to die, but she was more fearful of dying in a way that was unacceptable to her than of death itself. She was prepared spiritually for death. She had a clear vision of an afterlife, and she was very thankful for the high-quality time she had been able to spend with her husband and son. Finally, I double-checked my relationship with her family members to make sure that they could live with their role in Diane's passing.

In the final analysis, there was nothing left to negotiate. We were down to methods that would allow her to escape her suffering. Although society at present would prefer for Diane to have chosen to be medically sedated to unconsciousness to escape awareness of her suffering (see Chapters 12 and 13), she wanted no part of it. Dying sedated on a barbiturate infusion waiting for dehydration or sepsis to overcome her body made no sense to Diane. She would have found it humiliating, undermining all that she was trying to achieve. For Diane, a decisive end to her suffering at a time of her choosing by her own hand was very meaningful and in keeping with how she had tried to live her life. Sadly, she chose to be alone at the time that she took her overdose—not because she preferred to be by herself, but because she had researched the law in New York and had learned that anyone present at her death could be subject to potential prosecution. This is the part of her story I am least sanguine about. Although death was of her own choosing, no one should have to die alone; in these settings the laws prohibiting such acts simply do not make sense. Nevertheless, Diane died peacefully and secretly, by her own hand, as many others do in similar situations across the country.

Diane carved out a meaningful last phase to her complex life. Much of the richness of her last months stemmed from choices that she made in the context of medical decision making. Compared to the deaths of the preceding four acute leukemia patients who were treated at our hospital, Diane's course, though unconventional, was filled with meaning, joy, and human contact. Her choice of a purely palliative approach, eschewing the aggressive treatment that we so commonly and reflexively pursue, helped her make the most of her last months. The fact that she chose a hastened death at the very end, albeit by only a few days, in no way undermined the meaningfulness of the process. Since Diane had such well-developed fears about personal disintegration before death, her final three months was enhanced by the knowledge that there could be an escape if and when she needed it.

The Centrality of Partnership

Patients and their families have no choice about going through severe illness when someone is afflicted. Medical practitioners have the opportunity to give them the gift of partnership, which means to be both a professional adviser and also a friend and guide who is genuinely concerned about the patient's clinical course and outcome. Grappling in both a personal and professional way with the dimensions of illness outlined in Table 4–2 can help patients make good decisions in the face of overwhelming uncertainty. These decisions require an analysis of the medical facts that apply to the patient's condition, but should also take into account the patient's values and personal experience. Patients and their families also want medical professionals to use their own personal and professional experience to help guide the patient, and to make a commitment to care for the patient throughout the illness no matter where it goes.

Physicians and other health professionals who form these partnerships with patients and their families gain as much as or more than they give. They get an intimate glimpse at the human condition, and they have a rare opportunity to connect and make a difference. A physician's clinical and human skills are put to the test in these interactions, and working with a multidisciplinary team of skilled professionals, provides an opportunity for the physician to learn about him- or herself and about the power and limitations of medicine. Skills in forming and understanding partnerships get better with practice, and with every opportunity to care for articulate and challenging patients like Diane.

References

1. *Concise Oxford English Dictionary*, 7th ed. Oxford: Oxford University Press, 1982.
2. Quill TE, Brody H. Physician recommendations and patient autonomy: Finding a balance between physician power and patient choice. *Ann Intern Med* 1996; 125:763–769.
3. Lazare A, Eisenthal S, Frank A. Clinician/Patient Relations II: Conflict and Negotiation. In: Lazare A, editor. *Outpatient Psychiatry*. Baltimore: Williams and Wilkins, 1989.

4. Carrillo JE, Green AR, Vetancourt JR. Cross-cultural primary care: A patient-based approach. *Ann Intern Med* 1999; 130:829–834.
5. Catanzaro A, Moser RJ. Health status of refugees from Vietnam, Laos, and Cambodia. *JAMA* 1982; 247:1303–1308.
6. Kleinman A, Eisenberg L, Good BJ. Culture, illness and cure. Clinical lessons from anthropologic and cross-cultural research. *Ann Intern Med* 1978; 88:251–258.
7. The SUPPORT Principal Investigators. A controlled trial to improve care for seriously ill hospitalized patients. The study to understand prognoses and preferences for outcomes and risks of treatment (SUPPORT). *JAMA* 1995; 274:1591–1598.
8. Jones WHS. *Hippocrates*. Cambridge MA: Harvard University Press, 1923.
9. Quill TE, Dresser R, Brock DW. Rule of double effect: A critique of its role in end-of-life decision making. *N Engl J Med* 1997; 337:1768–1771.
10. Quill TE, Lo B, Brock DW. Palliative options of last resort: A comparison of voluntarily stopping eating and drinking, terminal sedation, physician-assisted suicide, and voluntary active euthanasia. *JAMA* 1997; 278:1099–2104.
11. Block SD. Assessing and managing depression in the terminally ill patient. ACP-ASIM End-of-Life Care Consensus Panel. *Ann Intern Med* 2000; 132:209–218.
12. Duberstein PR, Conwell Y, Cox C, Podgorski CA, Glazer RS, Caine ED. Attitudes toward self-determined death: A survey of primary care physicians. *J Am Geriatr Soc* 1995; 43:395–400.
13. Dickinson GE, Tournier RE. A decade beyond medical school: A longitudinal study of physicians' attitudes toward death and terminally-ill patients. *Soc Sci Med* 1994; 38:1397–1400.
14. Neumann JK, Olive KE, McVeigh SD. Absolute versus relative values: effects of medical decisions and personality of patients and physicians. *South Med J* 1999; 92:871–876.
15. Hamilton DG. Believing in patients' beliefs: physician attunement to the spiritual dimension as a positive factor in patient healing and health. *Am J Hospice Palliat Care* 1998; 15:276–279.
16. Kirschling JM, Pittman JF. Measurement of spiritual well-being: a hospice caregiver sample. *Hospice J* 1989; 5:1–11.
17. Ward J. A survey of general practitioners' attitudes to the involvement of clergy in patient care. *Br J Gen Pract* 1990; 40:280–283.
18. Lo B, Quill TE, Tulsky J. End-of-life Care Consensus Panel. Discussing palliative care with patients. *Ann Intern Med* 1999; 130:744–749.
19. Fisher R, Ury W. *Getting to Yes: Negotiating Agreement Without Giving In*. Boston: Houghton-Mifflin, 1981.
20. Quill TE. Principle of double effect and end-of-life pain management: Additional myths and a limited role. *J Palliat Med* 1998; 2:333–336.
21. Byock I. *Dying Well: The Prospect for Growth at the End of Life*. New York: Riverhead Books, 1997.

5

Nonabandonment: A Central Obligation
of Physicians

. . . the secret of the care of the patient is caring for the patient.
—Francis Peabody, 1927

Nonabandonment is a concept exemplified in a continuous caring partnership between physician and patient. This relationship may begin in health or in sickness, last through potential recovery or adjustment to chronic illness, and continue until a patient dies.[1-9] It acknowledges and reinforces the centrality of an ongoing personal commitment to caring and problem solving between physician and patient. Nonabandonment also captures the essential qualities whereby physicians and patients commit to mutual decision making over time, even when the course is uncertain. Many dimensions of this covenant are articulated in the virtues of caring, fidelity, altruism, and devotion,[10-13] yet none of them captures the particular importance of a long-term, engaged presence that continues until the patient dies or recovers.

Nonabandonment suggests a human relationship with an open-ended commitment over time. It is particularly mandated by three challenging aspects of modern medicine. One is the changing health care environment and its growing

An original version of this paper was co-authored by Dr. Christine Cassel, and published in the *Annals of Internal Medicine* 1995; 122:368–374.

emphasis on managed-care systems and competitive market approaches to cost containment. These forces may limit a patient's choice of physicians, disrupting the continuity of a physician–patient relationship by requiring frequent changes in exclusive provider organizations.[14] The growing prevalence of chronic illness and the aging of the population are other challenges that bring the centrality of nonabandonment into focus. For these populations, the evaluation of clinical performance must move beyond episodically making decisions about diagnostic or therapeutic options to establishing a relationship grounded in continuity, realistic expectations, and a shared understanding of goals and values. Finally, medicine's extraordinary success in prolonging life, as well as its ability to increase suffering and prolong dying if used indiscriminately, reinforces the importance of long-term committed medical relationships. Severely ill patients need physicians who will help them understand medicine's potential, given where they are in their lives' trajectories, and work with them through to their deaths to achieve the best possible quality and meaning in their lives. In this environment, making nonabandonment an essential obligation of all physicians seems vitally important. We focus our presentation with two clinical experiences.

Cynthia*

Cynthia was a 37 year-old graduate student in psychology. She was a practicing Buddhist who considered quality, human connection, and spirituality to be central to her life. She developed dyspeptic symptoms, and in three days her illness escalated from stress-induced gastritis to potentially treatable gastric lymphoma to terminal metastatic gastric adenocarcinoma.

Cynthia was devastated by her diagnosis. When her physicians recommended hospice care and promised to keep her free of pain until her death, she felt abandoned. She found no hope in their offer and needed to find a way to fight her illness. Although she understood the poor odds and potential toxic effects of experimental treatment, she believed she could beat the odds. Accepting her prognosis without a medical fight would have meant giving in to hopelessness and despair.

As Cynthia explored experimental therapy, she needed assurance that she could stop the treatment at any time if it became too harsh or was not working. She also needed to inquire about what dying might be like. She feared severe physical pain, lingering on the verge of death without

---

* Cynthia's story is presented in greater detail in Chapter 1 of *A Midwife Through the Dying Process: Stories of Healing and Hard Choices at the End of Life.* Baltimore: Johns Hopkins University Press, 1996.

quality of life, and being kept alive without sufficient consciousness. Because death in her religious tradition was a form of rebirth, she hoped that her physician would help her find death should she consistently experience any of these conditions, all of which seemed more terrifying to her than death itself.

To a physician with a belief in the hospice philosophy and negative feelings about the futile, medically invasive treatment of dying patients, Cynthia's request for an aggressive medical approach posed a significant initial challenge. Cynthia needed the slim hope that experimental medical intervention provided, but she also needed honesty about the odds and the potential toxic effects of such treatment. Armed with assurance that she would not be abandoned no matter what her clinical course, Cynthia eventually chose experimental therapy, despite its potential risks and burdens.

Not surprisingly, treatment was harsh and ineffective against the relentless progression of the cancer. As the burdens of her illness and its treatment increased, hospice care began to have a different meaning for her. The promise of intensive attention to symptom relief now seemed much more comforting than futilely fighting her disease. All subsequent efforts were directed to maximizing the quality of her time that remained. Because the tumor had invaded her entire abdomen, she depended on intravenous fluids and nutrition, which she chose to continue. A continuous intravenous morphine drip helped relieve her pain.

Cynthia went home with the support of her family and a home hospice program. She tried to find meaning in each day and simultaneously prepared for death. She married her longtime boyfriend, and her parents moved to town to be near her. The local Buddhist community had regular group meditations at her home. She gave away many of her favorite possessions as she prepared for death. It was an intensely sad and unforgettably meaningful time for all who had the privilege of being with her.

After several weeks, Cynthia's quality of life deteriorated despite everyone's best efforts. She required increasing doses of morphine, and she had to make hourly trade-offs between pain and sedation. She had nausea and vomiting that could not be relieved, and her wounds and ostomies had an unpleasant smell that she found inescapable and humiliating. Cynthia sadly accepted her inevitable death and said good-bye to the important people in her life. At this point, no viable avenues were available to recapture quality in her life, and further disintegration and suffering were larger enemies than death itself.

Because her physician had made a commitment not to abandon Cynthia at this critical moment, the physician's obligation was to help her find death on her own terms as much as possible. For Cynthia, this meant discontinuing central hyperalimentation treatment and accepting the sedation that came with escalating doses of the intravenous narcotics that were used to control her pain. She was prepared to die but did not want to be perceived as committing suicide. She and her family were reassured that this method was fully compatible with widely accepted ethical principles.

Cynthia gradually became more sedated, went into a coma, and died peacefully several days later, with her husband, parents, and friends in attendance.

Mrs. K.*

Mrs. K. is a 93 year-old woman who survived the Nazi death camps where most of her family had perished. She began a new life in the United States, raised one son in her second marriage, and outlived her husband by 20 years. She lives alone in a small apartment, and her social contacts are increasingly limited because of her own physical infirmities and the deaths of many friends.

She was healthy until eight years ago, when a painful neuropathy developed in her left leg. It was eventually diagnosed as reflex sympathetic dystrophy. Seeking pain relief and a way to stem its associated loss of strength, she saw an unending series of consultants. Trials of antidepressants, antiepileptics, nonsteroidal and narcotic analgesics, orthotics, and physical therapy were ineffective and often had unacceptable side effects.

She valued only two medications: flurazepam (Dalmane) for inducing sleep and diazepam (Valium) for treating the "aggravation" of chronic pain. Despite being very clear that these medications were helpful to her, Mrs. K. was repeatedly told by a series of physicians that these were the wrong medications because of their long half-lives, sedative side effects, and potential for addiction. Mrs. K. was determined to express her concerns, attributions, and experience to each physician she saw; she would dismiss most medical suggestions other than the two medications above as unworkable, and then proceed with her litany of problems—pain, sleeplessness, loneliness, and frustration from old age and infirmity. She was strong-willed and opinionated, and traveled from physician to physician to everyone's frustration.

After repeating this unproductive pattern of intervention and rejection, I eventually realized that what she needed most was to be cared about and listened to. I discovered that Mrs. K. did not expect medical answers to

* Mrs. K. was cared for by Dr. Christine Cassel, the coauthor on the original paper.

all of her problems. She wanted a confidante and adviser, someone who knew the whole picture and could interpret what was happening to her and find value in her personhood. I began to listen intently to her descriptions of the suffering and frustration of her daily life. Learning about her past suffering and losses in the death camps, and about how she survived, I came to understand how lonely it could be to outlive one's family and friends. Through this listening, Mrs. K. became more complex to me as a person, which allowed me to empathize more meaningfully with her plight. I helped her with bouts of constipation, guided her through cataract surgery, conservatively evaluated her chest pain of uncertain cause, and allowed her to openly explore whether life was worth living in the face of loneliness and loss. I also reinitiated therapy with flurazepam and diazepam without constantly questioning her need or their efficacy, accepting the small risk that she could be secretly stockpiling them in case she decided to end her life.

Although she remains lonely and frightened much of the time, Mrs. K. does not have to face the future alone. When she must confront medical challenges and even death in the future, she will have the distinct advantage of working with a medical guide who knows and respects her.

The Obligation of Nonabandonment

As shown in these two cases, the quality of medical care can be substantially enhanced when it is provided in the context of a caring, continuous, committed physician–patient relationship. The mutual decision making described in these two case presentations can never be adequately covered in formal "practice guidelines," treatment algorithms, or rigidly defined contracts. Standardized approaches cannot possibly attend adequately to the distinct and profound specificity of the patient and physician as persons or the shared experiences and meanings that develop between them over time. Medical care can be both humanized and individualized in such relationships. Respect for and curiosity about the person are essential[1,8] as is the desire to actively involve patients in their own care and empower them as much as possible.[7] Although patients often become more dependent and vulnerable when ill, a caring, committed relationship can respect and explore that vulnerability while allowing as much choice and control as possible given the patient's circumstance and personality. Relationships between physicians and patients can be both personal and professional, and empathy[15] and personal connection[9] can enrich the task of facing the reality of the patient's condition together.[16–18] Intuition and emotion supplement the intellect, and there is a flow between sharing information and making decisions about the patient's condition, while exploring any associated feelings and reactions.

The obligation of nonabandonment emphasizes the longitudinal nature of a caring and problem-solving commitment between physician and patient.[1,2,5,6,9] Principle-based ethical analyses of clinical actions sometimes focus on one moment in time and seek generalizable rules or answers. Patients and their families and physicians, however, do not have the luxury of existing in such isolation. Clinical decisions involve a series of choices over time, and the consequences of one decision may immediately and inevitably lead to a series of subsequent new dilemmas, each with its own cascade of consequences.

Furthermore, the meaning and critical nature of any particular medical act cannot be understood or judged by isolating it into rules that do not acknowledge the personal histories, values, motivations, and intentions of the persons involved.[10,11,19-24] For example, Cynthia's discontinuation of life-sustaining treatment at the end of her life had wide moral acceptance even though it resulted in a desired death (she was "allowed to die" of her underlying disease). Easing her death under these circumstances might be viewed as fulfilling a final commitment to not abandon her to further personal disintegration, which she had begun to view as worse than death. However, if that decision stemmed in part from under-treated pain, or from her physician's personal frustration with the difficulty of her dying, then such "allowing to die" could be the worst form of abandonment. Thus, any act cannot be fully understood or judged by putting it into an abstract category without considering the values, intentions, and circumstances of the actors.

Promising to face the future together is a central obligation of the physician–patient relationship.[1-9] This commitment is open-ended, for neither person knows what the future will hold nor what might be asked for or required. The American Medical Association (AMA) Council on Ethical and Judicial Affairs has stated a minimal expectation: "Once having undertaken a case, the physician should not neglect the patient, nor withdraw from the case without giving notice to the patient, the relatives, or responsible friends sufficiently long in advance of withdrawal to permit another medical attendant to be secured."[25] The depth and specificity of this obligation may vary from patient to patient, depending both on the patient's requests and clinical circumstances and on what the patient can and is willing to commit to. For me as Cynthia's physician, nonabandonment initially meant promising to work with her in a desperate fight against her disease but evolved to helping her find meaning, choice, and symptom relief as she faced death. For Dr. Cassel and Mrs. K., nonabandonment meant a willingness to share the patient's loneliness and suffering, acceptance of the limits of medicine, and staying alert for those opportunities when medical advice might improve her function, mood, or most recent crisis. For both Dr. Cassel and me, nonabandonment meant being there for our patients through the end of their lives, no matter what the clinical path.

The specific methods that these commitments eventually require cannot be known at the outset. Most physicians and patients commit to a process of working together through an unknown future. The physician is committed to responding to the patient's clinical situation and requests in an open-minded way, but is not obligated to violate his or her own values and beliefs in the process. When such conflict arises, the physician and patient should make every effort to find common ground and shared meaning. Mrs. K. and her physician eventually worked together in a way that allowed her to share her loneliness, report symptoms without having to be constantly tested, and procure an adequate amount of benzodiazepines without having to constantly justify her need. The meaning and morality of any clinical actions largely depend on the quality of mutual decision making, the depth of the interpersonal relationship, and the shared meaning that they reflect.

Nonabandonment reinforces several obligations for physicians when they encounter vulnerable persons and populations. At a societal level, physicians as professionals and as persons must help solve the problems caused by a lack of basic health care services and a coherent primary care system for disempowered segments of our community.[26-28] The continuity of care that we are committed to preserve in health care reform has never been widely available to the poor and uninsured. Many such persons are being abandoned to impersonal and episodic care only until their medical or psychosocial problems become so overwhelming that the medical system has no choice but to accept them.

Nonabandonment also reflects an obligation to respond to vulnerable persons whom we contact in our daily clinical work. Just as we must commit to working with the dying or chronically ill for whom cure is impossible, we must learn how to work with persons with overwhelming psychosocial and medical problems. This commitment does not imply an ability to resolve all such problems, but it does require that a physician be willing to care about, advocate for, and ultimately not desert such persons. A physician may be the only caring contact and advocate that many disadvantaged persons have.

Two Key Illustrations of Nonabandonment in End-of-Life Care

Although there are many times in the course of a severely ill patient's clinical course at which nonabandonment can be demonstrated, two are particularly important and illustrative.

Reassurance About the Future

Whenever a person is diagnosed with a potentially life-threatening illness, or when a clinical course takes a turn for the worse, he or she will begin to contemplate the future—including what dying and death might be like. Some-times, particularly late at night when usual distractions disappear, this imagi-native journey will take the patient to the deaths he or she has known or seen. If the person has witnessed harsh death, or death where physicians were not adequately responsive, the experience may well be frightening.

For Cynthia, given her Buddhist beliefs, her psychological and spiritual state as a person at the moment of death would have a strong bearing on how she would be reborn in the next life. Dying at peace bodes very well, whereas dying in agony might have devastating implications. For her, dying in peace meant being in control of her mental faculties, preserving alertness and the ability to connect with others, and not experiencing extremes of physical suffering. Mrs. K., on the other hand, survived the horrors of the Holocaust. How these memories influenced her search for relief from chronic pain and loneliness is not certain, but it is likely that such remembrances would come into her conscious awareness at times were she to be diagnosed with a terminal illness.

Fortunately, patients will talk about these fears and experiences if health care providers have the courage to ask about them. Questions such as "How have other people died in your family?" or "What are your biggest fears about the future?" often yield very important information about a patient's prior experiences with death and dying. When a patient reports witnessing a painful death where insufficient pain medication was provided, physicians should promise no such reluctance on their part. If the patient has seen severe shortness of breath or agitated delirium before death, it may not be easy for physicians to simply reassure. Most patients and families want their health care providers to be willing to face the unknown together with them, and to address any extremes of suffering that may arise. Most are less concerned with the methods of assistance than the willingness to work together until the patient's death. This commitment by one's physician and health care team is at the core of nonabandonment, and should be explicitly articulated whenever a patient's clinical course deteriorates significantly. Those patients and families who have this reassurance are more free to spend their precious psychic energy on other matters.

Responding to Extremes of Suffering

Patients who receive state-of-the-art palliative care delivered by a committed multidisciplinary team may develop symptoms at times in their illnesses, but most do not experience extremes of unrelieved suffering. Therefore, the physician's initial commitment will usually be satisfied by standard palliative care protocols and procedures. But some patients, like Cynthia, have good relief of symptoms for a time, only to experience more extreme suffering as death approaches. Fulfilling one's commitment to remain responsive and not abandon is critical at this time. When Cynthia's quality of life had deteriorated to the point where she was ready to die, it was clear, after a careful review, that our palliative approach was comprehensive but inadequate to sufficiently relieve her suffering. We then had to consider how best to help her. (The clinical approach to assessing such patients is reviewed in Chapter 9.) Once the team was assured that no opportunities for better palliation were being missed, the challenge was to help Cynthia find death in the least harmful way possible. The ways in which this might be accomplished are presented in Chapter 12. Cynthia was allowed to stop intravenous fluids and accept the sedation that would likely come with higher doses of analgesia. Fortunately, both of these interventions have widespread clinical, ethical, and legal support, so the process of easing her death was conducted out in the open with consensus building, consultation, documentation, and support. Contrast this with Diane's experience, described in Chapter 3. When Diane was facing a similar dilemma at the very end of her life, she had to be assisted in secret because the method she had chosen was illegal and more ethically controversial. In my opinion, the differences between the methods chosen in these circumstances are less critical than the careful clinical assessments, assurance of adequate palliative care, respect for the patient's values, and the commitment not to abandon.

Nonabandonment and Traditional Ethical Principles

Traditional ethical analyses often apply the principles of autonomy, beneficence, nonmaleficence, and justice to critical moments in medical decision making.[10,19] In this section, we explore how the obligation of nonabandonment might be integrated into and help inform these four principles.

The principle of autonomy focuses on a patient's right to have sovereignty over medical matters that pertain to his or her own body. In the United States, patients have a right to consent to or refuse potentially life-sustaining treatment and can have any treatment discontinued if it no longer meets their goals.[29-31] Cynthia initially had a right to both request experimental therapy and then later have treatment with intravenous fluids discontinued. A patient's request does not automatically obligate the physician to acquiesce. In fact, passively acceding to a patient request that defies the physician's recommendations and clinical judgment without fully informing the patient and actively exploring alternatives can be interpreted as a form of abandonment. Furthermore, the language of patient rights suggests that physicians have unrestricted obligations to patients, but physicians also have autonomous values and limitations that need to be respected. Ideally, patients will be given the opportunity to express their requests, hopes, and goals. The physician's responsibility is to seriously consider and try to respond to them without violating his or her own values. When there is conflict, a solution is of necessity a result of a negotiated agreement between autonomous partners, but it must also be based on a covenantal relationship of mutual respect and caring about the patient's best interests.[12,32,33] Autonomy gives each individual's self-determination its highest value, and may inadequately represent the central importance of the relationship and interpersonal connection that were at the core of Cynthia's and Mrs. K.'s treatments.

The principle of beneficence, as it applies to health care, means that a physician's actions are intended to benefit the patient; it is the principle most closely related to nonabandonment. Whether a given act is considered beneficent may depend on the nature of the act itself or on its meaning to the participants in the context of their relationship. Considered in the abstract, actively easing the death of a terminally ill patient who requests to die rather than continue to suffer can be considered either a compassionate act[5] or a fundamental violation of medical ethics,[34] depending on one's values and point of reference. Which constitutes abandonment—forcing Cynthia to continue to suffer against her will when a wished-for death is her only relief, or intentionally helping her to die? How does her Buddhist philosophy, with its emphasis on quality of life, connection, consciousness, and death as a form of rebirth, affect these considerations? How could Cynthia's physicians have acted beneficently if she had not been receiving a life-sustaining treatment that could be discontinued or if she had not had pain that justified increasing doses of narcotics? For Mrs. K., who suffers without the potential escape provided by a terminal illness, openly exploring the consequences of choosing death rather than continued living may be central to her search for meaning. Such explorations are often essential to good medical care, because they uncover ways in which a physician can help that do not involve actively assisting death.[35] However, exploring these domains with patients does not automatically include an obligation to accede to particular requests. We do not yet know what vexing ethical decisions will need to be faced in Mrs. K.'s future to fulfill the commitment not to abandon her—she knows only that she will not have to face these decisions alone.

The principle of nonmaleficence is captured in the maxim "above all, do no harm." Walking away from patients in severe need would clearly be harmful, but otherwise the specifics of what constitutes abandonment have been debated. The choice that committed physicians and their dying patients face is sometimes among competing "harms"—is it worse to directly or indirectly assist suffering patients to achieve a wished-for death, or to force them to continue to suffer against their will? The "bright line" between "allowing to die" and "causing death" can become indistinct when physicians are faced with real patients who are suffering intolerably and to whom they have made a commitment of nonabandonment. Such a commitment at least calls for creative solutions so physicians can stay within their value structure and still help their patients in need. Two recently proposed solutions—barbiturate sedation to treat uncontrollable suffering,[36] and allowing patients to stop eating and drinking to achieve a wished-for death,[37,38]—are presented in Chapter 12. Although such solutions may stretch the boundaries of rule-based medical ethics, avoidance of disintegration and humiliation before death requires that we consider innovative solutions to fulfill our obligations.[36-40] Because honesty and truth telling are so critical in these delicate deliberations, the clinician's intentions in these matters should be clarified as much as possible.[41]

The principle of justice asks us to look beyond the individual to the aggregate good of society when considering a particular policy. The effects of any individual clinical act on the community and the profession must also be considered, even in the face of overwhelming individual suffering. In the health care reform movement, nonabandonment would focus our attention on the 43 million people who are currently uninsured, many of whom live in poverty. How can we justify spending hundreds of thousands of dollars of public funds on individual persons for unproven therapies when we are not providing even basic health care, nutrition, and shelter for major segments of our society? When we consider changing public policies to avoid abandoning the dying, we must consider both the individual persons who would be helped and the potential effect on other vulnerable populations. Perhaps facing death more boldly with our patients would enhance overall medical care at the end of life and add personal meaning to physicians' work, thus reclaiming the moral base of the profession.[5,39] It is also possible, however, that such policies would promote our society's penchant for seeking quick fixes for complex moral and medical problems.[34,42] Nonabandonment should always focus our attention on the most vulnerable persons and groups, and would encourage health care professionals to struggle on their behalf.

The ethical discourse that emanates from these four principles can be abstract, analytical, and impersonal, where preset positions and theory are given prominence over the complex stories of actual persons. The obligation of nonabandonment can enrich this analysis by asking us to always consider the particular commitments and circumstances of each patient and physician, who are doing their best to make decisions together in the patient's best interests given the uncertainties of the patient's condition. General policies and rules must find room for patients who are facing unique circumstances.

New Ethical Paradigms

Exciting new theoretical frameworks have emerged in an attempt to remedy the problems created by too rigid an application of ethical principles. These models are relevant to the principle of nonabandonment. The glimpse of them provided in this section does not do justice to their richness and complexity, but the interested reader can explore them further using the references provided. In analyzing medical dilemmas, these schools of thought place particular emphasis on the importance of the particular persons involved, their relationships with one another, the many levels of meaning and intention in their work together, and the processes of their interaction and decision making.

Casuistry, for example, asks us to apply ethical principles to the understanding of particular cases, and to not always focus on universal or generalizable implications.[22] Analyzing particular cases only from the perspective of pre-existing positions tends to keep the discussion abstract, superficial, and impersonal. Casuists ask us to grapple with actual cases, and in doing so make the analysis better reflect clinical realities. For example, how does Cynthia's Buddhist faith, which places utmost importance on dying with inner spiritual peace, bear on the physician's responsibility to respond when her suffering became extreme toward the very end of her life? How might the response have been different for Christian patients for whom otherwise analogous suffering had a completely different meaning, potentially putting them closer to God? The meaning of autonomy, beneficence, and nonmaleficence each could vary with the personal values, spiritual background, and clinical circumstances of the patient.

Clinical narratives that reflect the "lived experience" of physicians, patients, and families add layers of depth and feeling to the discussion.[43,44] Through narratives, we often learn more about the multidimensional nature of human life— that intention, emotion, and meaning are textured, contradictory, and much more complex than ordinary rule-based ethics acknowledge. The clinical narrative about Diane presented in Chapter 3, which was published in the *New England Journal of Medicine* in 1991,[45] helped to change the debate about whether it could ever be morally justified for a physician to actively help a patient to die. Prior to that time, the only real cases discussed in the public domain had been those of Jack Kevorkian, and those stories were so dominated by his bizarre personality and unusual methods that they were easy to dismiss.[46] Diane's story, presented as a clinical narrative without apology or explanation, forced readers to put a more human face on the patient and physician, and more carefully consider the potential moral place of physician-assisted death as a last resort in the context of a caring relationship.

Phenomenologists remind us that there are no objective observers or reporters of these processes—the best we can do is acknowledge our biases and try to understand and be explicit about how we interpret and translate reality.[23,47] Phenomenologists also warn us against reducing lived experience to simple rules, theories, or moral maxims and exhort us to try to remain true to the particular persons grappling with the dilemma. Thus, readers of this book

must analyze my ostensibly objective presentations and analyses of clinical situations with the knowledge that I am an advocate of both hospice care as the
standard of care for the dying and of the possibility of a physician-assisted
death as a last resort. I also believe strongly that such actions should be carried
out only in the context of a long-term doctor–patient relationship, and that
patients should have a strong and central voice in all of their medical decisions.
The stories that I am likely to select for presentation, the medical experiences
I am likely to have, and the manner in which I choose (both consciously and
unconsciously) to present them may be biased in that direction. Readers must
make up their own minds in determining if these biases interfere with or add
to the arguments.

Feminist ethics highlights the importance of caring and of relationships—
that kindness, mercy, empathy, devotion, altruism, love, and generosity have
central roles in medical ethics that are often not adequately reflected in principles.[24,48] These qualities, so central to understanding real-life experience, are
usually not included in principle-based ethical analyses. The fact that I had
known Diane for many years before her terminal diagnosis, and that we had a
deep personal relationship as a result of shared medical experiences, may have
had a bearing on my willingness to take a professional risk on her behalf toward
the end of her life. Had we been strangers, or had Diane been less articulate
about her needs, it might have been more difficult for me to argue that I was
basing my responses on my commitment not to abandon her. In addition,
feminist ethics underscores the importance of community, and warns of the
danger of sexual bias, domination, and subordination, which may occur subtly
or explicitly. How might the fact that Diane was a female patient interacting
with a male physician have influenced our decision making? Were these socio-
cultural factors overshadowed by Diane's clarity about what she needed, the
fact that her request was consistent with deeply held personal values, and my
long-standing commitment to keep patients' values in the forefront of medical
decision making? The potential of having medical decision making influenced
in such unconscious ways is one of the most powerful reasons for bringing very
challenging life-and-death decisions out into the open, to seek consultation
from those with special expertise, and to achieve consensus among those who
care about the patient.

Cross-cultural ethics reminds us that the meaning of an act may vary not only
with the persons involved but also with the culture within which the persons
live.[21] "Generalizable" rules derived by a particular ethicist may in fact unconsciously reflect his or her sex, culture, and preexisting biases and experiences;
thus, such "objective" analysis and even principles chosen as fundamental
should be open to scrutiny and viewed from a culturally relative perspective.
Thus, we may have widely differing views about not only the controversial issue
of physician-assisted death[34,49] but also differences in using or not using feeding

tubes[50,51] or other potentially life-sustaining treatments. Even in matters as seemingly noncontroversial as hospice care, we find a significant underrepresentation of African Americans and other minority groups.[52-54] Since hospice care is felt to be the standard of care for the dying, this disturbing trend deserves exploration and understanding. It may stem from the historical reality of being deprived of access to basic health care, or a lack of trust in a medical system potentially withholding effective treatment, or a cultural bias in favor of preserving life no matter how much suffering exists, or other factors. The cultural factors that influence access to and delivery of palliative care services clearly warrant further exploration and research.

According to virtue ethics, acts cannot be understood without acknowledging and exploring the inner character and motivation of the actors.[11] Like rule-based ethics, virtue ethics looks to the meaning and intention of the participants. Yet instead of trying to fit real human intentions into finely drawn, abstract ethical rules, virtue ethics explores in depth the complex motivation and quality of interaction between the specific clinician and patient around a particular act. Thus, in trying to understand and evaluate Cynthia's final decision to accept sedation and stop her life-sustaining intravenous feeding, a virtue ethicist would ask that one look beyond the particular type of act (both of these acts have wide social and legal acceptance). The fact that Cynthia was prepared for death to come sooner rather than later was important in this decision, as was her Buddhist belief in rebirth and the importance of dying without extremes of suffering at the end. The facts that I was helping her to die at her request, that I understood that she was ready, and that for me the methods of assistance were relatively unimportant would also need to be considered. My objective was to fulfill the commitment to Cynthia that I had made several months earlier—that I would be responsive if her suffering became harsh. Virtue ethics would try to explore and integrate this complexity in an effort to evaluate the morality of a particular act.

Through each of these alternative ethical paradigms runs the assertion that general principles must be applied in the context of relationships between particular persons with unique histories and commitments to one another. These ethical analyses include consideration of the potential closeness between physician and patient, strong feelings of caring and connection, a willingness to take risks on behalf of one another, and a promise not to abandon no matter what the future holds. Seemingly logical principle-based ethical distinctions sometimes lose their sharpness in the context of such relationships, as commitments and obligations supersede abstract principles. Nonabandonment is a central obligation in these relationships. It evokes less abstract but no less theory-based associations to genuine patient and family experiences than principles of autonomy, beneficence, nonmaleficence, and justice.

By reemphasizing the centrality of the physician–patient relationship in medical ethics, a balanced tension between individual decision making and more general ethical considerations can be made more explicit. For example, my obligation to ease Cynthia's death in a manner acceptable to her and her family when her personhood began to disintegrate seemed to override my obligation to make sure that any contribution to her death be inadvertent and unintentional. This latter requirement is derived from the rule of double effect (explored in Chapter 11), a complex and somewhat controversial moral doctrine derived from Roman Catholic theology that is strongly represented in Western medical ethics. Yet the rule had little or no meaning in this context for either Cynthia or me as her physician. It was, however, important to Cynthia that she find a way to die that would not be considered "suicide." Fortunately, we were able to find an acceptable way for her to die that was responsive to her clinical condition and acceptable to her as a person. Although Diane also found a way to die that was acceptable to her as a person and responsive to her clinical condition, the method she required was incompatible with current legal mores. Therefore, the process went underground, and she felt forced to die alone to protect her family from potential legal repercussions. Medical ethicists frequently over-emphasize the method of assistance and under-emphasize the quality of caring, commitment, and joint decision making that led to these acts. No one should have to die alone because of abstract, impersonal ethical principles or arbitrary legal prohibitions.

Limitations of Nonabandonment

The central commitment of nonabandonment as an obligation of physicians must be balanced by other ethical considerations.[55] Although physicians should try to respond to the needs and requests of their patients over time, they should not violate their own values in the process. A creative tension should exist between respect for the values and choices of unique human beings, on the one hand, and respect for societal traditions, precedents, and more general implications on the other. Thus, there should always be a dynamic interplay between patient and physician, individuals and society, traditional and personal values, subjective interpretations and objective analysis, and emotion and intellect. Grappling with these inherent tensions should add depth and complexity to the moral decision-making process and thus more accurately reflect the reality of the human condition.

Nonabandonment as an obligation has inherent limitations. Beyond a basic notion of ensuring some form of continuity as suggested by the AMA, the depth and nature of this commitment may vary for both physician and patient. The relationship is partly defined and explicit, but partly open-ended and implicit, more of a covenant than a contract.[12,32,33] Although the focus of this chapter has primarily been on the obligations of physicians, these relationships are ultimately reciprocal if not equal or symmetrical. Often, the rewards for physicians who make these commitments far exceed what is required of them, but the extent of caring and the level of personal responsibility will ultimately depend on a mutual give-and-take with the patient over time. Sometimes, as with my relationship with Cynthia, the pace of coming to know one another is accelerated by a severe illness. At other times, the depth of a relationship is limited by either party's reluctance or inability to trust or to address major medical issues (for example, substance abuse or dementia). Through shared experience over time, a comfortable and effective level of interaction that ranges from superficial to intense can usually be established with the patient or the patient's surrogates.

Although many clinicians choose the profession of medicine because of their need to serve and care, they must also lead balanced, healthy lives.[56] Many clinicians are more skilled at recognizing and responding to the needs of others than their own needs.[57] If we ask clinicians to provide a more caring, long-term commitment to their patients, we must also reinforce their need to set limits and take care of themselves. For physicians, these limits might be expressed by limiting practice size, or encouraging group practice for the built-in support system and potential of shared coverage. Although fully committed relationships are clearly ideal, given the complexity and diversity of patients and doctors, the possibility of limited relationships under some circumstances, or even explicit termination when a mutually satisfactory relationship cannot be established, must be allowed. There is sometimes an unresolvable tension in medicine between the commitment to the care of others and commitment to self-care.

We must also try to ensure that our ethical precepts and our health care system reinforce rather than undermine clinicians' willingness to engage with patients when their problems seem insoluble or are not clearly resolved by current ethical thinking. The principle of nonabandonment is paramount and may allow clinicians to take some risks on behalf of patients who have no good alternatives. Clinicians, however, should not violate their own fundamental values simply because a patient requests a certain kind of assistance. Clinicians' personal values should be explored and challenged but ultimately respected. A clinician should make every effort to find common ground with such a patient, and to find alternative ways of responding. Such analyses often require intense self-examination and consultation with trusted colleagues. We must try to both challenge and respect our limitations.

Concluding Thoughts

Nonabandonment is fundamental to the long-term physician–patient relationship, as well as to other relationships between clinicians and their patients.

Patients seek clinicians who will make a commitment to both care about and know them as persons, and to be guides and partners in sickness and health until their deaths. In this context, clinicians and patients can learn to judiciously use the power of medicine and expand the concept of healing to include working with persons with severe chronic illness and disability and those who are dying. A commitment not to abandon supplements a caring relationship because it requires that the clinician and patient work together over time, even when the path is unclear. Clinical and moral challenges must be met and engaged with the patient, not shied away from by recourse to falsely bright lines or unbending rules. There is a world of difference between facing an uncertain future alone and having a caring partner who will be present no matter what happens.

Such commitments between clinicians and patients are at the core of the medical profession, so they must be explicitly represented in the discourse of medical ethics. Physicians who find that their work with patients has lost its excitement and meaning would do well to consider whether they are engaged in these types of relationships. Health planners, legislators, risk managers, medical educators, and ethicists should carefully examine whether their contributions to health care tend to reinforce or obstruct such commitments. Clinical medicine is ultimately a humbling and exhilarating profession, filled with joy, sorrow, and an overabundance of uncertainty that comes with establishing a genuine long-term connection with patients. To practice medicine with a commitment to caring and being present and responsive no matter what the future holds is to experience the richness of the human condition over and over again and to know one has made a difference. If the obligation of nonabandonment is better incorporated into medical ethics, medicine may become more humanized and more responsive to the real problems faced every day by physicians and patients.

References

1. Peabody FW. The care of the patient. *N Engl J Med* 1927; 88:877–882.
2. Cassell EJ. *The Nature of Suffering and the Goals of Medicine*. New York: Oxford University Press, 1991.
3. Frankl VE. *Man's Search for Meaning*. Boston: Beacon Press, 1959.
4. Buber M. *I and Thou*. New York: Charles Scribner's Sons, 1937.
5. Quill TE. *Death and Dignity: Making Choices and Taking Charge*. New York: W.W. Norton and Co., 1993.
6. Subcommittee on Evaluation of Humanistic Qualities in the Internist. A guide to awareness and evaluation of humanistic qualities in the internist. Portland, Oregon: American Board of Internal Medicine 1985 (available upon request).
7. Novack DH. Therapeutic aspects of the clinical encounter. *J Gen Intern Med* 1987; 2:346–355.

8. Rogers CR. *On Becoming a Person: A Therapist's View of Psychotherapy*. Boston: Houghton-Mifflin, 1961.
9. Matthews DA, Suchman AL, Branch WT Jr. Making "connexions": Enhancing the therapeutic potential of patient-clinician relationships. *Ann Intern Med* 1993; 118:973–977.
10. Beauchamp TL, Childress JF. *Principles of Biomedical Ethics*. New York: Oxford University Press, 1994.
11. MacIntyre A. *After Virtue*. Notre Dame, Indiana: University of Notre Dame, 1984.
12. May WF. *The Physician's Convenant: Images of the Healer in Medical Ethics*. Philadelphia: Westminster Press, 1983.
13. Ramsey P. *The Patient as Person: Explorations in Medical Ethics*. New Haven: Yale University Press, 1970.
14. Emanuel EJ, Brett AS. Managed competition and the patient-physician relationship. *N Engl J Med* 1993; 329:879–882.
15. Zinn W. The empathic physician. *Arch Intern Med* 1993; 153:306–312.
16. Lidz CW, Appelbaum PS, Meisel A. Two models of implementing informed consent. *Arch Intern Med* 1988; 148:1385–1389.
17. Katz J. Duty and caring in the age of informed consent and medical science: unlocking Peabody's secret. *Humane Med* 1992; 8:187–197.
18. Quill TE, Townsend P. Bad news: Delivery, dialogue and dilemmas. *Arch Intern Med* 1991; 151:463–468.
19. Johnson AR, Siegler M, Winslade WJ. *Clinical Ethics: A Practical Approach to Ethical Decisions in Clinical Medicine*, 2nd ed. New York: MacMillan, 1986.
20. Toulmin S. The tyranny of principles. *Hastings Cent Rep 2000*; 11:31–39.
21. Gustafson JM. Moral discourse about medicine: A variety of forms. *J Med Philos* 1990; 15:125–142.
22. Jonsen AR, Toulmin S. *The Abuse of Casuistry: A History of Moral Reasoning*. Berkeley, CA: University of California Press, 1988.
23. Zaner RM. *The Way of Phenomenology*. New York: Bobbs-Merrill, Inc., 1970.
24. Sherwin S. *No Longer Patient: Feminist Ethics and Health Care*. Philadelphia: Temple University Press, 1992.
25. American Medical Association Council on Ethical and Judicial Affairs. (1986). *Current Opinions—1986*. Chicago: American Medical Association.
26. Noble J, de Friese GH, Pichard FD, Meyers AR. Concepts of health and disease. In: Noble J, editor. *Textbook of General Medicine and Primary Care*. Boston: Little, Brown, 1987; 3–13.
27. Showstack J, Fein O, Ford D, Kaufman A, Cross A, Madoff M, et al. Health of the public: the academic response. Health of the Public Mission Statement Working Group. *JAMA* 1992; 267:2497–2502.
28. Kraut AM. Healers and strangers: Immigrant attitudes toward the physician in America—A relationship in historical perspective. *JAMA* 1990; 263:1807–1811.
29. President's Commission for the Study of Ethical Problems in Medicine and Biomedical and Behavioral Research. (1983). Deciding to forgo life-sustaining treatment: A report on the ethical, medical and legal issues in treatment decisions. Washington, DC: U.S. Government Printing Office.
30. American College of Physicians. *American College of Physicians Ethics Manual*. *Ann Intern Med* 1992; 3d(117):947–960.
31. American Medical Association's Council on Ethical and Judicial Affairs. Decisions near the end of life. *JAMA* 1992; 276:2229–2233.

32. Quill TE. Partnerships in patient care: A contractual approach. *Ann Intern Med* 1993; 98:228–234.
33. Emanuel EJ, Emanuel LL. Four models of the physician-patient relationship. *JAMA* 1992; 267:2221–2226.
34. Gaylin W, Kass LR, Pellegrino ED, Siegler M. "Doctors must not kill." *JAMA* 1988; 259:2139–2140.
35. Quill TE. Doctor, I want to die. Will you help me? *JAMA* 1993; 270:870–873.
36. Troug RD, Berde DB, Mitchell C, Grier HE. Barbiturates in the care of the terminally ill. *N Engl J Med* 1991; 327:1678–1682.
37. Eddy DM. A conversation with my mother. *JAMA* 1994; 272:179–181.
38. Bernat JL, Gert B, Mogielnicki RP. Patient refusal of hydration and nutrition: An alternative to physician-assisted suicide or voluntary active euthanasia. *Arch Intern Med* 1993; 153:2723–2727.
39. Quill TE, Cassel CK, Meier DE. Care of the hopelessly ill. Proposed criteria for physician-assisted suicide. *N Engl J Med* 1992; 327:1380–1384.
40. Sedler RA. The constitution of hastening inevitable death. *Hastings Cent Rep* 1993; 23:20–25.
41. Quill TE. The ambiguity of clinical intentions. *N Engl J Med* 1993; 329:1039–1040.
42. Singer PA, Siegler M. Euthanasia—a critique. *N Engl J Med* 1975; 292:78–80.
43. Brody H. *Stories of Sickness*. New Haven: Yale University Press, 1987.
44. Hunter KM. *Doctors' Stories: The Narrative Structure of Medical Knowledge*. Princeton: Princeton University Press, 1991.
45. Quill TE. Death and dignity: A case of individualized decision making. *N Engl J Med* 1991; 324:691–694.
46. Cassel CK, Meier DE. Morals and moralism in the debate over euthanasia and assisted suicide. *N Engl J Med* 1990; 323:750–752.
47. Baron RJ. An introduction to medical phenemenology: I can't hear you while I'm listening. *Ann Intern Med* 1985; 103:606–611.
48. Gilligan C. *In a Different Voice: Psychological Theory and Women's Development*. Cambridge: Harvard University Press, 1982.
49. Brock DW. Voluntary active euthanasia. *Hastings Cent Rep* 1992; 10–22.
50. Sullivan RJ. Accepting death without artificial nutrition or hydration. *J Gen Intern Med* 1993; 8:220–224.
51. Gillick MR. Rethinking the role of tube feeding in patients with advanced dementia. *N Engl J Med* 2000; 342:206–210.
52. Rhymes J. Barriers to effective palliative care of terminal patients. *Clini Geriatr Med* 1996; 12:407–416.
53. Tong KL. The Chinese palliative patient and family in North America: A cultural perspective. *J Palliat Care* 1994; 10:26–28.
54. Crawley L, Payne R, Bolden J, Payne T, Washington P, Williams S. Palliative and end-of-life care in the African American community. *JAMA* 2000; 284:2518–2521.
55. Pellegrino ED. Compassion needs reason too. *JAMA* 1993; 270:874–875.
56. Quill TE, Williamson P. Healthy approaches to physician stress. *Arch Intern Med* 1990; 150:1857–1861.
57. Miller A. *Prisoners of Childhood. The Trauma of the Gifted Child and the Search for the True Self*. New York: Basic Books, 1981.

6

Delivering Bad News

MRS. JOHNSON: "I feel as if I've been robbed of a future."

A 37 year-old man who used intravenous drugs was diagnosed with human immunodeficiency virus (HIV). He and his wife were estranged and had not had sexual relations in three years. His wife, Mrs. Johnson, was an independent, family-oriented, devoutly Christian, African-American woman with three children. She worked as a nurse's aide. In the past, she had a prolactin-secreting pituitary adenoma for which she had reluctantly and intermittently accepted medical treatment (bromocriptine). She generally preferred to be treated exclusively by her faith in God, taking the medication only when her prolactin level became so elevated that her breasts released large amounts of milk. She and I had known each other for six years, and our recurrent complex discussions resulted in a close relationship wherein each of our perspectives was understood and respected by the other.

When her husband was diagnosed with HIV, Mrs. Johnson came to see me to discuss her situation and assess her risk. We discussed the available diagnostic tests and the difference between HIV (even without treatment, patients can carry the virus for many years without major medical problems) and AIDS (a more advanced state of illness characterized by immunologic vulnerability to unusual infections). She understood the distinction, but she continued to equate any infection with AIDS. She decided she wanted to be tested, but when asked what she would do if her test was positive, she responded, "I don't know, but I don't think God would do this to me." The conversation left me unnerved, but we went ahead with the test and planned a follow-up visit to discuss the results.

The results showed that she was HIV infected. I felt sad for her as a person, and was also unsettled as I realized for the first time that the epidemic was truly reaching all walks of society. I also began to dread our meeting where I would deliver the bad news. I was uncertain how she would respond, and feared the results could shake the foundations of her faith (one of her major strengths) and her sense of who she was. What follows is an unedited transcript of the first minutes of our meeting when the bad news was shared.

MRS. JOHNSON: *Is it bad?*

DR. QUILL: *I'm afraid it is.*

MRS. JOHNSON: *Oh no, Dr Quill. Oh my God!*

DR. QUILL: *I was shocked too.*

MRS. JOHNSON: *Oh God. Oh Lord have mercy. Oh God, don't tell me that. Oh Lord have mercy. Oh my God. Oh my God, no, Dr. Quill. Oh God. Oh no. Please don't do it again. Please don't tell me that. Oh my God. Oh my children. Oh Lord have mercy. Oh God, why did He do this to me? Why did He do this to me? Why did He do this to me, Dr. Quill? Oh Lord have mercy. Oh my God, Jesus.*

DR. QUILL: *You're still all right at this point, okay.*

MRS. JOHNSON: *You don't know how long I've had it, Dr. Quill?*

DR. QUILL: *I don't know.*

MRS. JOHNSON: *I can't sit.* (She paces around the room.)

DR. QUILL: *It's okay.*

MRS. JOHNSON: *Why did he do this to me? Why? What have I done to him? Why does he do this to me? Why? Why? Why? Oh Lord. What am I going to do with all of my children? I won't be able to see my grandchildren. I just had another grandbaby. I won't ever be able to see . . . I won't live to see the baby. I won't be able to get up off my chair. Oh, Dr. Quill, I don't know what to do. Oh God, I don't know what to do. My son-in-law is not going to let the kids come over.*

DR. QUILL: *First thing we have to do is learn as much as we can about it, because right now you are okay.*

MRS. JOHNSON: *I don't even have a future. Everything I know is that you gonna die anytime. What is there to do? What if I'm a walking time bomb? People will be scared to even touch me or say anything to me.*

DR. QUILL: *No, that's not so.*

MRS. JOHNSON: *Yes they will, 'cause I feel that way about people. You don't know what to say to them and what to do. Oh God.*

DR. QUILL: *What we have to do is learn some things about it . Even though it's scary, it may not be as scary as you think. Okay?*

MRS. JOHNSON: *Oh my God. Oh my God. I hate him. I hate him. I hate the ground he walks on. I hate him, Dr. Quill. I hate him. He gave this to me. I hate him. He took my life away from me. I have been robbed. I feel as if I have been robbed of a future. I don't have nothing.*

DR. QUILL: *There is a future for you.*

MRS. JOHNSON: *They don't even have a cure for me.*

DR. QUILL: *There's a lot of work going on right now, and you can have the infection for a long time before you get sick. There is a lot of research going on.*

MRS. JOHNSON: *I read about it. I have a friend with it. I went over to the university . . . Since you told him [her husband] he had AIDS, he has been at my house and I feel so sorry for him. I was being nice to him. Oh my God, my God. It just doesn't pay to be nice. It doesn't. What do you get out of it?*

DR. QUILL: *Neither you nor he knew that there was a risk back then.*

MRS. JOHNSON: *Another cross to bear.*

DR. QUILL: *You never did anything wrong.*

MRS. JOHNSON: *What am I going to tell my children when they are old enough to tell them?*

DR. QUILL: *Before you tell them anything, you are going to learn a lot about this.*

MRS. JOHNSON: *I can't go home. I can't even stay here. I'm so scared. Oh my God. I knew that you were going to tell me this. I always liked you. I didn't want you to tell me this. Oh God. I don't know if I can deal with this. I don't know, Dr. Quill, if I can deal with this.*

DR. QUILL: *You've worked through this before. It's going to be hard, but it may not be as bad as you think. Okay? I think what you have to do . . .*

MRS. JOHNSON: *I got my church, Dr. Quill. I can't let them see me like that. I can't do it. I would rather . . . because I can't let our church see me like this. They mean a lot to me. Oh, Dr. Quill, and my daughter. Oh, I won't see my daughter and my baby.*

DR. QUILL: *You are still the same person. Okay?*

MRS. JOHNSON: *Why is He doing this to me?*

DR. QUILL: *I don't know. You are still the same person. What you have to do is eventually learn as much as you can about this. The odds are that you are going to stay healthy for a long time. Okay? You are still very healthy right now.*

MRS. JOHNSON: *What you telling me? I still have a chance to beat it? Can I beat it?*

DR. QUILL: *I think that is possible.*

MRS. JOHNSON: *How can you be sure when you don't even know what the cure is for it?*

DR. QUILL: *A couple of things, okay? We don't think you've had this very long; a couple of years at the most. All right. A lot of people believe that the virus can stay around for many years before it produces many problems. Sometimes six or eight years. There is a lot of research going on now to try to find ways to treat it.*

MRS. JOHNSON: *Oh God, Lord Jesus.*

DR. QUILL: *You may have a lot of time before we have to deal with this. I think the first thing we have to do is probably get some further blood tests. We should, because it's such a surprise for you and for me that you have it, even though we think we know how you got it. We maybe should repeat it to be a hundred percent, a thousand percent sure,* even though they repeat it once. I think that's wise to do, because the only way that you could have gotten it is from your husband. I think we ought to repeat it even though we know that it is probably true.

MRS. JOHNSON: *I don't know if I can live with myself . . . in my bed right now. I don't like him, Dr. Quill. I don't even want to stand by him. I won't even stay with him. I won't. Why must I pay for his sins? Why?*

DR. QUILL: *There's nothing fair about it.*

MRS. JOHNSON: *My children.*

DR. QUILL: *It's very scary. Also, there are a lot of things we can do.*

MRS. JOHNSON: *Oh Lord have mercy. Then I have the pituitary thing.*

DR. QUILL: *Like your pituitary tumor, it has been there for years. It doesn't . . .*

MRS. JOHNSON: *It's not the same.*

DR. QUILL: *No, it's not the same thing. If the tumor gets worse, we know what the treatment is.*

MRS. JOHNSON: *It's not the same. It can't be cured. You talking about something they never came up with, never came up with a cure for. I've got nothing. All they can do is just treat whatever comes along, like a cold, or pneumonia, stuff like that—that's all.*

DR. QUILL: *That's right. But right now there are millions and millions of dollars being poured into research, and that's what we have to hope for.*

MRS. JOHNSON: *It doesn't make me feel good.*

DR. QUILL: *I wish I had something more clear to tell you, but I think there are a lot of folks who are in the same shoes that you're in and they are all hoping. They are figuring out ways to cope. That's what we have to figure out.*

MRS. JOHNSON: *Dr. Quill, will you still be my doctor?*

DR. QUILL: *Absolutely, I will.*

MRS. JOHNSON: *You promise?*

DR. QUILL: *Absolutely. We'll meet very regularly so we know what's going on.*

MRS. JOHNSON: *Okay, all right. I'm so scared. I don't want to die. I don't want to die, Dr. Quill. Not yet. I know I got to die, but I don't want to die.*

DR. QUILL: *We've got to think about a couple of things. . . .*

We both felt overwhelmed by the news and the encounter. With great difficulty, I allowed her rage and terror to be expressed, yet I also clumsily attempted to find some boundaries to her experience. I was concerned that she would lose the ability to cope, and I needed to be reassured before she left the office that she envisioned a basic plan. It was also not completely clear whether it was her or me that I was trying to protect. Through the intense emotional expression, she raised several basic questions that needed to be addressed: (1) Am I still the same person? (2) When am I going to die? (3) How contagious (repulsive) am I? (4) Will you still be my doctor? (Will I be alone?) (5) How can I tell my family, friends, and church? Though these questions were by no means simple, struggling to answer them began to give some definition to her problem.

My struggle to respond adequately caused me to reflect on the process of delivering bad news. In spite of the fact that all clinicians regularly conduct interviews where bad news is shared, there is little descriptive medical literature,[1-7] even less research,[8] and almost no formal training in medical school or residency about how to do it.[9] Although the medical literature is limited, useful information can be extracted from psychology literature describing responses to overwhelming stress[10-12] and crisis intervention.[13,14] Using this literature, combined with videotape material and role-playing of the actual delivery of bad news, I have conducted experiential workshops with expert clinicians and trainees to learn about their beliefs and strategies. The schema presented herein represent a synthesis of these data, incorporating my own clinical experience both as a general internist and a palliative care physician. This chapter emphasizes the initial delivery of bad news, when a patient is first coming to grips with a new problem, rather than needs and strategies that evolve over time.

Background

Bad news can be defined as anything that drastically and negatively alters one's view of oneself as a person, and of one's future. An initial diagnosis of HIV or of a potentially lethal cancer certainly qualifies for most individuals. Even though effective treatments may be available, one's self-image as a healthy person is clearly threatened. Because of our faith in the power of medical treatments to thwart disease, clinicians are often tempted to focus immediately on the efficacy of treatment, without exploring the devastation that such news entails. Yet our job must begin by responding to the personal meaning of the loss and its attendant emotions, and then eventually connecting the experience with the potential hope of effective treatment and/or palliation. Although I struggled repeatedly to do this in the interview with Mrs. Johnson, my initial efforts to find boundaries and offer hope were premature and ineffective. My responses probably stemmed in part from my own difficulty in tolerating such painful emotions associated with hopelessness (*"I feel as if I have been robbed of a future. I don't have nothing."*), as well as my desire to help Mrs. Johnson to feel better. Eventually, after she had expressed her devastation more fully, Mrs. Johnson was able to begin to hear some very simple versions of the fact that treatment was available, and that the news was not quite as bad as she had thought.

Patients bring to a discussion their own set of experiences and preconceived notions about a particular illness with which they are faced, giving them a unique frame of reference. For Mrs. Johnson, a diagnosis of HIV was a death sentence (*"I won't live to see the baby."*) associated with progressive debility (*"I won't be able to get up off the chair."*) and social ostracism (*"My son-in-law is not going to let the kids come over."*). It takes time and energy for me as a clinician to first understand these beliefs more fully and then respond to them in ways that are both honest and hopeful. My premature efforts at reassurance, though at times awkward and ineffective (*"It may not be as bad as you think."* ... *"You are still the same person."* ... *"The odds are you are going to stay healthy for a long time."*) may have been useful and important in that they planted seeds of hope that eventually could lead to increased understanding. They also demonstrated that my view of this disease was not the same as hers, and that the two could perhaps be reconciled in the future.

Sometimes a patient is devastated by what seems to the clinician to be a minor diagnosis, such as mild high blood pressure. When a patient responds to a new diagnosis with strong emotion, the clinician might ask, "What is the most frightening part?" or "What experiences have you had with high blood pressure in the past?" before offering reassurance. Perhaps high blood pressure is associated with a devastating stroke in one of the patient's parents, or with kidney failure in a close friend. Once this experience has been explored and understood, the clinician can begin to reassure the patient that blood pressure is usually readily responsive to treatment, and if treated, complications can usually be avoided. Reassurance can thus be tailored to the patient's particular fears. Other times, a clinician may learn that a patient is in the midst of major marital problems and sees the diagnosis as emblematic of the "pressures" he or she have been under at home and at work. Sorting out this complex mixture of psychosocial and biomedical components of the patient's blood pressure is central to its eventual treatment, but understanding what contributes to the initial response to bad news is the first step. Since the meaning of any bad news is highly individual, the initial exploratory interview is very important to set the proper foundation for personalized treatment.

Two critical elements are present in successful bad news interviews: (1) creating a therapeutic dialogue based on carefully listening to the patient's experience, beliefs, and reactions, and (2) imparting guidance and information tailored to the patient's circumstances and needs. Sometimes a new, medically important diagnosis does not even qualify as bad news to a particular patient in the sense that he or she is not threatened as a person, nor does his or her future feel threatened. For example, perhaps everyone in a patient's family has hypertension, and all have been treated without complication. Learning that one has high blood pressure might be expected, and lead directly to asking the clinician for a recommendation, resulting in a simple transaction about behavioral and pharmacological interventions. Thus, each bad news interview must begin with careful observation of verbal and nonverbal cues that may suggest important personal meanings a new diagnosis might have for the patient.

Medical diagnoses, especially those that are genuinely life threatening, can transform a person's self-concept from that of someone who is well with a full future to that of someone who is sick with a shortened life span. This capacity for bad news to powerfully and, initially at least, negatively transform a person's self-image is one of the reasons it is so difficult to do. Even when patients know that the news is not going to be good, later they can often recall the moment when they got the final diagnosis, including the exact wording. In Mrs. Johnson's case, the devastation was inherent in the news. A different technique of bad news delivery would not have made it less emotionally charged. My search to find some way to reassure her did not lessen the loss. Perhaps it might have been better to simply explore her experience in all its enormity and try to empathize with her. Later, after she had been more fully heard and acknowledged, she was more receptive to reassurance. ("It's very scary. Also, there are a lot of things we can do.") She would probably not have been able to listen to the "things we can do" earlier, and it might have been perceived as not listening to or minimizing her experience.

There are barriers on all sides that impede the delivery of bad news. Patients do not necessarily want to hear news that has the potential to adversely affect them as persons, and physicians do not want the power that their knowledge and words can have under these circumstances. In hopes of softening the impact, physicians sometimes use ambiguous language subject to misinterpretation—such as the word "tumor" rather than "cancer." Furthermore, physicians are trained to treat diseases and tend to be enthusiastic about promising treatments, but they are less well prepared for handling associated emotions and integrating a person's beliefs and experiences into a treatment plan. With increasing pressure to shorten hospital stays and reduce treatment plans according to predetermined algorithms that are disease-driven, there is even less time to allow patients to personally integrate bad news before embarking on treatment. Reimbursement plans do not cover the time needed to meet with a patient and family, to fully consider the diagnosis, and to make sure decisions are made based on a full understanding of options. Whether they are covered by a reimbursement plan or not, these exchanges remain vital to high-quality patient care.

Although these barriers make the delivery of bad news a challenging endeavor, systematic approaches have been developed to aid clinicians who understand the fundamental importance of this process to patient and family well-being. In the next section, I explore some of crucial elements in the successful delivery of bad news, and then I offer a practical approach to the actual interview. This will be followed by outcomes that might be expected from an initial interview that is conducted successfully.

Advance Preparation

Advance knowledge about a patient's strengths, weaknesses, and coping style can be invaluable in deciding how to present bad news. Mrs. Johnson's spiritual beliefs, support from her children, and fierce independence were clearly her strengths. Her previous fearful, ambivalent feelings and denial about medical diagnosis and treatment of her pituitary adenoma were potential sources of concern. Our discussions concerning her knowledge and beliefs about HIV allowed her to begin anticipatory grief work. They also allowed me, as her physician, to begin to understand the potential meaning of the news to her. Her view regarding what she would do if infected (*"I don't know, but I don't think God would do this to me"*) was ominous, and I should probably have explored it in more detail before delivering the diagnosis.

The physician is usually the first to get any kind of medical news. Particularly if there has been a close physician–patient relationship in the past, the physician may have to grieve him- or herself before meeting with the patient and family. My own sad feelings over Mrs. Johnson's condition prompted me to seek out one of my close colleagues and explore my own reactions to the news before proceeding. It was useful to fully experience my own grief before I encountered hers. It is also incumbent on the physician to make sure that the information about a diagnosis is accurate and that he or she is knowledgeable about its medical implications, including prognosis and further treatment options. If a patient has a condition with which the physician is unfamiliar, the physician must learn enough about it to be informative and to be able to answer general questions about prognosis and therapeutic options in this initial meeting.

Bad news, particularly that which has the potential to be devastating to the patient, should be delivered in a face-to-face encounter in a private setting, with time set aside to allow for questions. The patient should be offered the option of having close family members attend the meeting, both for support and to serve as an added set of eyes and ears. Delivering bad news is generally not a task to be delegated or done in an indirect way, such as over the phone. However, there may be exceptional circumstances, such as an unanticipated new finding, that dictate some of the news be disclosed in this way. Although Mrs. Johnson did not want to come to the office to hear the news, the significant medical risk posed by the HIV diagnosis and the meaning she attached to the diagnosis made a face-to-face appointment mandatory. I encouraged her to bring along a close family member, or perhaps someone from her church, but she insisted on coming alone so she could hear the news privately, and then decide how to share it. Advance plans about how and when to share the news learned at a meeting are helpful, as are considerations of how directly or indirectly to involve significant others. Since Mrs. Johnson doubted that God would do this to her, we might have been well-served by a hypothetical conversation about what it might mean to her spiritually if she had HIV. *("What would it mean to you if the test is abnormal?")* Of course, even such a discussion does not guarantee that the subsequent bad news conversation will be any less devastating.

Frequently, questions are raised by physicians or families as to whether a patient is medically or psychologically strong enough to handle bad news.[5,6] Although there may be exceptional circumstances under which delivering bad news directly to the patient should be delayed or avoided, they require careful analysis of the question, Who is really being protected? For example, in some Hispanic and Russian cultures, bad news is frequently shared primarily with the family and not the patient. Contrary to the usual approach in the United States, where a premium is placed on patient autonomy, in these and other cultures it is considered cruel and inappropriate to tell a patient about bad news directly. Yet if the patient is competent, even if he or she is from a culture where patients are bad not told diagnoses, some advance assessment of the patient's preferences should be made. A patient's direct request to be told the diagnosis usually creates an obligation to do so that takes precedence over a family member's or a physician's fear of doing the patient harm, unless the clinical evidence suggesting possible harm is very persuasive. In other words, it is generally not the physician's role to protect a patient from the truth about his or her condition or from the ensuing grief. Exploring the family's fears and concerns, and discussing the necessity of responding truthfully to a patient's request to be told the diagnosis, may allow the family to better prepare for the moment their loved one is told. This discussion may be justified in the interest of overall patient and family well-being, provided the patient's condition is not likely to worsen significantly in the meantime.

Delivering the News

Robert Buckman developed a protocol for the delivery of bad news. It is summarized, with some modifications, in Table 6–1.[7] In describing each of these steps, I will outline some general concepts, then illustrate them with examples drawn from Mrs. Johnson's interview.

Greet and Calibrate

Careful attention should be given to the setting of a bad news interview. Whenever possible, such encounters should be made in a private setting. Ample time should be set aside for an in-depth exploration of whatever emerges in

TABLE 6–1. Initial Steps in Delivering Bad News

1. Greet and calibrate
2. Find out how much the patient knows
3. Find out how much the patient wants to know
4. Share information tailored to the individual
5. Respond to the patient's feelings
6. Make a plan and follow through

the conversation. Those family members whom the patient has brought and any clinicians who are present, should be given room to sit down, so that all are seated at the same level. As with all such encounters, the interview should begin with introductions of everyone present. The patient's immediate condition is an important starting point. If the patient is in severe pain or is overwhelmed with anxiety at the outset of the encounter, then these conditions should be explored and addressed before proceeding with the delivery of the diagnosis.

Some medical circumstances are so pressing that decisions must be made immediately. A patient who has suffered an acute heart attack cannot delay thrombolytic therapy or angioplasty without serious consequences. In this instance, some steps of the protocol must be compressed, and the physician must progress to the treatment phase more rapidly than would otherwise be ideal. Once the patient has stabilized, the clinician should revisit those steps that were given short shrift to make sure that the impact of the diagnosis on the patient has been understood, and that the patient is fully informed about the medical aspects of the decisions that have been made.

Mrs. Johnson and I met at a scheduled time in a private setting. Although we greeted as we usually did—by shaking hands—and sat down together, she began with a direct question *("Is it bad?")*. She knew the answer by looking at my face. Therefore, we were into the core of the bad news from the outset, based on her lead rather than mine. Delaying this exchange until we had had more time to get settled would have been inappropriate. On the other hand, having a physician jump right into such a conversation before the patient has given a clear indication that he or she is ready is also inappropriate, and might even be considered cruel. Thus, unless the patient requests the news, it is generally better to begin with a few minutes of exploration about how the patient and family have fared since the last visit. This is more than small talk. It allows the clinician, patient, and family a few minutes to get adjusted to one another, and to get emotionally prepared for the meeting. Those present can usually detect that the news is not good from the appearance and other nonverbal cues of the clinician (and there would be no need for such an adjustment period if the news were good). Nevertheless, there is an important difference between knowing that the news is bad and actually hearing it.

Find out How Much the Patient Knows, and How Much the Patient Wants to Know

An initial assessment of what the patient has been told or figured out, and her readiness to hear the news, are suggested initial steps. Mrs. Johnson requested the results as soon as I walked into the room, and she could read the answer on my face. Such explicit requests for information should be responded to directly, using clear, simple language that is comprehensible to the patient. Ideally, the specific language used has been defined in advance —perhaps when the purpose of the test was being explored. The complex associations of meaning that a person may have for words such as *tumor, cancer, malignancy, HIV infection,* and *AIDS* mean that mutual understanding is not a certainty at this point.

Other patients do not want to hear the news right away, or perhaps would rather not hear it at all. With these patients, time initially spent exploring how they are feeling, how they have fared since the test was taken, and what thoughts and feelings they have had about the test and about getting the results is extremely important. It allows the patient to control the flow of information and to have time to settle and brace him- or herself before hearing the news. It also helps the physician understand more about the patient's coping style and about the potential impact the news will have once delivered. Unless a patient specifically requests not to hear the news (a request that itself needs in-depth exploration and understanding), the physician eventually should deliver the news in a clear, sensitive manner. If the clinician gets the feeling that the time is right, he or she might signal the patient by asking, "Are you ready to hear about the test results?" Again, the patient probably knows that if the news were good, it would have been delivered quickly.

Share Information Tailored to the Individual Patient

If the news to be delivered has complex ramifications, the physician should avoid the temptation to deliver too much of it all at once. Each piece of news, from the reality of the diagnosis to its implications, may or may not have a profound impact on the patient. The patient should be given time and opportunity to respond. This is particularly true initially, when the patient's self-image and worldview may be severely threatened.[10,15] Though the patient's beliefs about a disease and previous reactions to stressful situations may help in predicting his or her response, this prediction is not always reliable, particularly if the news is perceived by the patient as overwhelming.

When surveyed well after receiving bad news, patients and families reported wanting a lot of information about the disease (prognosis, further tests, treatment options), reassurance about the physician's availability, and an opportunity to explore the impact of the disease on themselves, their families, and their careers.[16,17] Whereas all of these domains are important, information must be tailored initially to the patient's perception of the problem, to direct patient requests, and to correcting unrealistic views about the illness. Reconciling discrepancies between Mrs. Johnson's perception of HIV as a death sentence and medical realities about HIV's responsiveness to treatment and the likelihood of a significant latency period before her illness became symptomatic was a vital early informing task. Since the patient's initial ability to integrate information may be limited, the physician should give simple, focused bits of information, using language that the patient can understand. Both verbal and nonverbal responses to each piece of information should be attended to, and the amount of information conveyed should be keyed to the patient's continued active engagement. Unfortunately information-laden physician soliloquies can alienate the patient without truly educating.

The information Mrs. Johnson needed to hear at her initial visit included the following: (1) HIV infection usually has a long latency period, and there are medical interventions to help control it (there is hope); (2) she was contagious only through blood or sexual contact; (3) I would be her doctor and available to her; (4) she needed to tell her closest, most trusted supporting people, in this case her children; and (5) I would see her and any family she might choose in a few days. More complex information about HIV infection and its treatment, unless specifically requested, would probably not have been retained by the patient at this initial visit.

The physician, too, has informational needs. The physician must assess and respond to the patient's immediate risks from the diagnosis. Mrs. Johnson was not at significant risk from the biological effects of her disease, which were at an early stage. Her risk of being psychologically devastated, and potentially committing suicide, was significant. There is epidemiologic evidence of an increased incidence of suicide in individuals with AIDS[18,19] and other devastating illnesses, such as Huntington's chorea,[20] renal failure,[21] and cancer.[22] A mandate for early HIV counseling, support, and suicide assessment for those who test positive for the virus is supported by several anecdotal reports of suicide upon hearing a diagnosis.[23] Defining suicide risk in those with newly diagnosed, serious medical problems includes assessing suicidal thoughts, feelings, and intentions in the context of the patient's previous mental health or substance abuse problems, considering prior suicide attempts, and evaluating available social supports.[24-26] In a high-risk situation, experienced counselors, social support programs, the immediate involvement of significant others, and even short-term hospitalization are options. Suicide attempts immediately upon hearing bad news, before a patient has had time to fully integrate and under-stand its meaning, indicate the hopelessness, isolation, and desperation many patients initially feel.

To expect an initial interview of this kind to fully inform about a diagnosis, prognosis, and treatment plan is unrealistic. In Mrs. Johnson's case, because of the devastating effect of the news, and because there was no pressing medical need for immediate intervention, the informational goals of the encounter were scaled down dramatically. She learned she had HIV and that the disease was not as immediately dangerous or contagious as she had thought. Rather than focusing on treatment options, we needed to spend our energy achieving a common perception of the problem and its prognosis, and making a plan for telling her family and utilize her support systems. Before she left the office, she was able to assure me that she had no intention of ending her life, and that she was planning to inform her children and would call me in two days.

Respond to the Patient's Feelings

Mrs. Johnson reacted to her diagnosis of HIV as a profound threat to her as a person. Her response was based on her perception of and experience with HIV, which in many ways were not congruent with medical reality.[2,3,10,11] Her mis-perceptions needed to be recognized and sensitively worked on as part of cre-ating a healing partnership. Her belief that HIV was a death sentence, a disease that could transform her into a pariah, was overwhelming. ("*I don't even have a future. Everything I know is that you gonna die anytime. What is there to do? What if I'm a walking time bomb? People will be scared to even touch me or say anything to me.*")

Each perception had some truth and some distortion. The challenge for the clinician is to respond empathically to the patient's devastating feelings and perceptions, and at the same time try to correct distortions so that the emotional impact of the news has some boundaries and coping can begin. With Mrs. Johnson, emotions initially flowed freely. My job as her physician was to allow them to be expressed fully, while keeping a sharp eye out for opportunities to reconcile her perceptions with mine. Other patients' emotions may be too shameful or threatening to be openly expressed. In these circumstances, the physician might encourage their expression by asking "What is the most frightening part?" in an effort to understand the patient's inner experience.

When the threat of a diagnosis is severe, basic coping responses fall into three categories:[2,3,10,11] (1) basic psychophysiologic, (2) cognitive, and (3) affective. These are summarized in Table 6–2. The two basic psychophysiologic mecha-nisms for coping are the fight-flight response and the conservation-withdrawal response,[18] which correspond to activation of the sympathetic and parasympa-

TABLE 6-2. Coping Responses to Bad News

CATEGORY	EXAMPLES	
Basic psychophysiologic	Fight-flight	
	Conservation-withdrawal	
Cognitive	Denial	Disbelief
	Blame	Acceptance
	Intellectualization	
Affective	Anger	Shame
	Fear	Relief
	Anxiety	Guilt
	Helplessness	Hopelessness

thetic nervous systems, respectively. Mrs. Johnson exhibited the fight-flight response. She wanted to flee, and she began pacing around the small examination room, unable to sit still. I wanted to give her enough space, but I was also fearful that if she fled she might harm herself or find herself completely alone without any direction when this high-energy state wore off. Because she was allowed to pace and express herself, she was eventually able to accept personal support and information that helped put her losses in perspective, and we were able to devise a basic plan for follow-up.

Becoming withdrawn and silent upon hearing bad news is an example of the conservation-withdrawal response. Cognitive processes in this state are very limited, so patients often report feeling numb and having little recollection of the content of discussions beyond the initial bad news. In more extreme forms of this reaction, heart rate and blood pressure drop, and a patient who does not lie down may faint (vasovagal or neurocardiogenic syncope). In other species, this response has considerable value as a survival mechanism in threatening situations ("playing possum"). Expectations with respect to information exchange have to be scaled down considerably once a patient enters a conservation-withdrawal state.

There are five basic cognitive coping strategies: denial, blame, intellectualization, disbelief, and acceptance. Mrs. Johnson used denial as a cognitive coping strategy when she was diagnosed with a pituitary adenoma. It allowed her to lead a full, untroubled life without treatment in spite of substantial chronic leakage of milk from her breasts (galactorrhea).[27,28] When she was confronted with her HIV diagnosis, her initial cognitive responses were somewhat disorganized but were dominated by blaming her husband and God. She did not overtly express guilt, but she did openly wonder how this could happen to her after she had led such a good Christian life.

The cognitive response that physicians are most comfortable with is intellectualization.[6] Many patients (often to the relief of their physicians) seek information to control the emotional impact of their diagnosis. The physician should respond forthrightly to requests for information, but he or she should be aware that complex information may not be retained,[29] in part because of the patient's underlying affective state and the consequent cognitive disorganization caused by the news. If a patient's questions and quest for information become overly aggressive, they may represent an indirect expression of anger or blame that may need more exploration.

Disbelief occurs when patients hear a diagnosis but can't quite believe that it applies to them. Many patients initially experience this cognitive reaction upon hearing bad news. Some patients for whom disbelief is more persistent may ask to be repeatedly retested, or may seek second and third opinions. Disbelief is a close cousin to denial, though in the latter response thoughts about the illness are frequently kept out of cognitive awareness, whereas with disbelief, such thoughts are omnipresent. Finally, acceptance occurs when the bad news has been fully integrated into one's sense of person and plans are being made for moving forward. Complete acceptance sometimes takes considerable time and effort for patients to develop, and often a partial acceptance coexists along with several of the other cognitive reactions.

Affective responses are also present when anyone receives bad news. These may include anger (rage), fear (terror), anxiety, helplessness, hopelessness, shame, relief, or guilt. In Mrs. Johnson's case, the overwhelming affects were overtly expressed, whereas with other patients they may be hidden to the patient, the physician, or both. Mrs. Johnson's initial affects were consistent with the fight-flight response, involving a mixture of rage, terror, and fear. Feelings flowed, giving tremendous power to her cognitive responses and a frightening dimension to having her world and self-image under siege: *"Oh my God. Oh my God. I hate him. I hate him. I hate the ground he walks on . . . He gave this to me. I hate him. He took my life away from me. I have been robbed. I feel as if I have been robbed of a future. I don't have nothing."* Other patients may become acutely anxious or be dominated by feelings of helplessness ("There is nothing I can do") or hopelessness ("There is nothing anyone can do"). In comparison to Mrs. Johnson, other patients' affects may be much more subtle or covert. Nevertheless, if left unaddressed, these affects can exert a powerful influence on the patient and family, and can alter a patient's ability to cope effectively with his or her illness.

A patient's initial cognitive and affective responses must be explored before substantial efforts at patient education and informed decision making can proceed.[1,10] The depth of this exploration will depend on the strength of the patient's responses, the medical necessity for rapid decision making, and the physician's interpersonal skills. If a physician is unable to undertake this task, it should be delegated to a skilled person who has knowledge about the disease and experience working with patients.

To understand and respond to a patient's initial responses and distortions, the physician must listen, acknowledge, legitimize, explore, and empathize; these communication skills are described in detail elsewhere.[30-32] Exploring, listening to, and tolerating the patient's response to bad news are perhaps the most vital steps. To begin to relieve a patient's suffering, the physician must thoroughly understand the patient's unique experience of pain and the meaning of the loss. This is particularly difficult when part of the patient's response is anger and some of the blame is focused directly or indirectly on the physician. Feelings of hopelessness and despair also may be hard for physicians to tolerate, particularly when a patient has a condition that does not respond well to biomedical intervention. By hearing and attempting to understand and empathize with a patient's pain and struggle, the physician can help the patient feel less alone and therefore less overwhelmed, perhaps creating a foundation on which the patient can begin to face the problems ahead.

Not all patients will respond initially with cognitive distortions or strong affective responses. Some will simply want to know the medical facts and make prompt decisions. A patient who has been suffering with an undefined illness may actually feel relieved by bad news that at least clarifies the problem. By exploring the meaning that the news has for the patient, the physician can better understand whether an effectively neutral exchange of information represents a coping style (intellectualization) that helps control and limit affect, or in fact the news has little adverse meaning for the patient. Other patients will go elsewhere to work through the emotional side of their responses (family, friends, other health professionals), preferring to keep the physician–patient relationship a more traditional biomedical exchange.

Planning and Following Through

Being alone and isolated with a serious disease can cause severe suffering[1] and therefore should be avoided as much as possible. In Mrs. Johnson's situation, my continued presence as her physician no matter what the future held was one of the most important outcomes of the initial encounter. Her perception of HIV as shameful and dangerous led her to ask if I would still be her physician. After I reassured her about our relationship, our next step was to decide whether and how she could confide in her children and close family members. I offered to meet with her and her children at any time to address their concerns and questions. She eventually benefited from written material about HIV and AIDS, although this was more than she wanted in the initial encounter. Because of the overwhelming nature of her initial visit, it was premature then to talk about further medical staging of her disease or about initiating medical treatment; these would be addressed over the next several weeks and months. Fortunately, her disease did not require immediate intervention, or we would have had to try to push forward in spite of the difficulties.

Deciding how to work with Mrs. Johnson's fundamentalist Christian church was more complex. Her church viewed AIDS as God's response to sinful behavior. She decided it was too risky to share this information with her pastor, thereby losing a potentially important means of support. She was informed about the availability of help from support groups, social agencies, and several more receptive pastors, but Mrs. Johnson was reluctant to share her grief with strangers. Supports need to be mobilized at many levels, but always tailored to the individual patient.

The physician, too, may have support needs, particularly when the patient has a strong, sustained emotional response and/or when a patient's prognosis is very poor.[6] Physicians may also need advice about making difficult medical choices when the direction is still unclear after the medical facts and the patient's preferences have been explored thoroughly. These dilemmas are particularly difficult when there is a strong, long-standing physician–patient bond and a physician is experiencing his or her own grief. The support of trusted colleagues, physician support groups, or therapists can be extremely helpful for the physician, who should not suffer alone in this process either.

Desired Outcomes of Early Meetings

Desired outcomes of early meetings are summarized in Table 6–3. They include the following:

TABLE 6–3. Desired Outcomes of Early Meetings

1. Minimize aloneness and isolation
2. Achieve a common perception of the problem
3. Address basic information needs
4. Address immediate medical risks, including risk of suicide
5. Respond to immediate discomforts
6. Ensure a basic plan for follow-up
7. Anticipate what has not been talked about

Minimize Aloneness and Isolation

This simple yet profound outcome represents much of what needs to occur in the early meeting. Fully exploring the patient's emotional pain and cognitive responses, offering a continued presence, and mobilizing the patient's social supports are all part of this process. Social supports should be tailored to the individual patient, leaving the patient ultimately in control of who gets informed and involved. Physicians may also need to avail themselves of social supports to work through their own grief.

Achieve a Common Perception of the Problem

Understanding and exploring commonness and differences sets the stage for a deeper understanding of the meaning and implications of the news.[4,33] The physician's medical view of the problem needs to be reconciled with the patient's unique perception and personal implications. This process of understanding and exploring the patient's worldview can create a deep bond between the patient and physician, help alleviate isolation, and create a basis on which to build future mutual decisions.

Address Basic Information Needs

Information must be tailored to the needs of the individual patient. It should be straightforward and translated into terms the patient can fully understand. Information should be shared in small increments, with an opportunity for exchange on each point, rather than in a soliloquy. The physician should solicit and respond to a patient's questions and concerns. Complex educational objectives need to be achieved progressively, in many steps over time.

Address Immediate Medical Risks, Including the Risk of Suicide

The risk of suicide upon hearing a devastating diagnosis is significant, and should be carefully assessed in early meetings. Sometimes a medical situation increases the need for a patient to integrate bad news, but usually time can be allowed for integration before major medical decisions are made. When an approach is unclear, additional resources and opinions should be sought from knowledgeable people. Allowing time for the patient and physician to make proactive, informed decisions about a treatment (or nontreatment) can make a tremendous difference in the patient's attitude in participation, and in the outcome of the treatment.

Respond to Immediate Discomforts

If anxiety, restlessness, or insomnia are persistent and overwhelming, then a short course of anxiolytic medication may be indicated. Similarly, physical pain can be treated with analgesics while options to approach the underlying disease are being explored. The physician should make every effort to lessen severe emotional and physical discomfort using medical measures and interpersonal skills, but it should be kept in mind that some emotional pain is inevitable as a patient attempts to come to grips with bad news. If medications are to be used, they should be given in limited amounts because of the lability of the clinical situation and the potential risk of suicide. Discomfort that persists should be treated aggressively to minimize suffering.

Have a Basic Plan for Follow-Up

Having a basic plan for follow-up makes the physician's continued presence a reality and can alleviate a patient's sense of aloneness with the problem. A plan for informing and involving the patient's significant others should also be developed. It is advisable, particularly if the patient is feeling overwhelmed and out of control, to prescribe some concrete tasks: telling specific people, seeing a consultant, talking to individuals with similar problems, and/or writing down questions.

Anticipate What Has Not Been Talked About

If an initial meeting is all information and no affect, tell the patient he or she may have some strong feelings or reactions, and that they will be useful to talk about in future meetings. If the initial meeting is dominated by powerful emotional reactions, as with Mrs. Johnson, say that there may be many questions about the disease that can be discussed at future visits. A balanced process of affective exploration and information gathering that builds on a patient's perceptions and beliefs will help the patient begin to cope with bad news and make good decisions about future care.

Epilogue

When I spoke with Mrs. Johnson two days after our initial visit, she was in conversation with her family and had a few specific questions about her diagnosis. When she subsequently returned for a follow-up appointment, she was in a completely different psychological state. Her children could not have been more supportive, and they were more knowledgeable about the disease than she had anticipated. She had obtained written information from a community AIDS center that reinforced the optimistic picture that I was painting. She had specific questions about her disease and treatment options. She initially refused antiretroviral medical therapy, preferring to rely exclusively on her religious faith, although later in her illness she accepted a multidimensional approach that included medications.

As predicted, Mrs. Johnson remained healthy for several years before her immune system began to fail. She became subject to opportunistic lung and brain infections. Over time, we unfortunately had to have several more "bad news" conversations as her medical condition and prognosis deteriorated. None of these conversations was as emotional or devastating as the first, but they illustrate that for patients with severe progressive illnesses, there are a series of losses over time, often marked by discrete transitions punctuated by the exchange of bad news. The potential for devastation as well as the opportunity for reintegration are present at each transition.

I am extremely grateful to Mrs. Johnson, whose initial struggle is so graphically described in this chapter, for her generosity in sharing her experience. Throughout her illness, her children were a source of great joy and support, as was her religious faith, though she never shared information about her illness with her church members. As death approached, she had frequent opportunistic infections that necessitated hospitalization, but she was able to spend most of her time at home cared for by her family. She eventually died with AIDS dementia. She and her family have given many of us lessons about courage and resiliency. Her story is chronicled more completely in a book chapter titled "Another Cross to Bear."[34]

- *Note*: The dialogue and some of the associated commentary in this chapter were originally presented in a manuscript I published along with my wife, Penny, titled "Delivering bad news: dialogue, delivery and dilemma," *Archives of Internal Medicine* 1991; 151:463–468.

References

1. Cassell EJ. The nature of suffering and the goals of medicine. *N Engl J Med* 1982; 306:639–645.
2. Myers BA. The informing interview: enabling parents to "hear" and cope with bad news. *Am J Dise Children* 1983; 137:572–577.
3. Hoy AM. Breaking bad news to patients. *Br J Hosp Med* 1985; 34:96–99.
4. Goldie L. The ethics of telling the patient. *J Med Ethics* 1982; 3:128–133.
5. Reiser SJ. Words as scalpels: Transmitting evidence in the clinical dialogue. *Ann Intern Med* 1980; 92:837–842.
6. Zinn WM. Doctors have feelings too. *JAMA* 1988; 259:3296–3298.

7. Buckman R, Kason Y. *How to Break Bad News: A Guide for Health Care Professionals. Baltimore*: The Johns Hopkins University Press, 1992.
8. Walsh RA, Girgis A, Sanson-Fisher RW. Breaking bad news 2: What evidence is available to guide clinicians? *Behav Med* 1998; 24:61–72.
9. Yieing D, Kjein RE. Delivering the bad news: The most challenging task in patient education. *Am Optom Assoc* 1987; 58:660–663.
10. Jewett LS, Greenberg LW, Champion LA, et al. The teaching of crisis counseling to pediatric residents: A one-year study. *Pediatrics* 1982; 70:907–911.
11. Lazarus RS. *Psychological Stress and Coping Process*. New York: McGraw-Hill International Book Co., 1966.
12. Cohen P, Lazarus RS. Coping with the stress of illness. In: Stone GC, Cohen P, Adler NE, editors. *Health Psychol* San Francisco: Jossey-Elms, 1979, pp. 217–254.
13. Kubler-Ross E. *On Death and Dying*. New York: MacMillan, 1969.
14. Jacobson G, Stricker M, Morley WE. Generic and individual approaches to crisis intervention. *Am J Public Health* 1968; 58:338–343.
15. Cassell EJ. *The Nature of Suffering and the Goals of Medicine*. New York: Oxford University Press, 1991.
16. Novack DH. Therapeutic aspects of the clinical encounter. *J Gen Intern Med* 1987; 2:346–355.
17. Weisman AL, Worden WJ. (1980). Report of Project Omega: coping and vulnerability in cancer patients. Massachusetts General Hospital, Harvard Medical School.
18. Marzuk PM, Tierney H, Tardff K, Gross EM, Morgan EB, Hsu MA. Increased risk of suicide in persons with AIDS. *JAMA* 1988; 259:1333–1337.
19. Frierson RL, Lippmann SB. Suicide and AIDS. *Psychosomatics* 1988; 29:226–231.
20. Farrer LA. Suicide and attempted suicide in Huntington's disease: Implications for preclinical testing of persons at risk. *Am J Med Genet* 1986; 29:226–231.
21. Abram HS, Moore GL, Westervelt FB. Suicidal behavior in chronic dialysis patients. *Am J Psychiatry* 1971; 127:119–124.
22. Louhivuori A, Hakama M. Risk of suicide among cancer patients. *Am J Epidemiol* 1979; 109:59–65.
23. Faulstick ME. Psychiatric aspects of AIDS. *Am J Psychiatry* 1987; 144:551–556.
24. Whitlock PA. Suicide in physical illness. In: Hoy AM, editor. *Suicide* Baltimore: Williams and Wilkins, 1986, pp. 151–170.
25. Hatton C, Valente S. *Suicide: Assessment and Intervention*, 2nd ed. East Norwalk, CT: Appleton & Lange, 1983.
26. Hall JM, Stevens PE. AIDS: A guide to suicide assessment. *Arch Psychiatr Nurs* 1988; 1:115–120.
27. Suchman AL, Matthews DA. What makes the patient–doctor relationship therapeutic? Exploring the connectional dimension of medical care. *Ann Intern Med* 1988; 108:125–130.
28. Watson M, Greer S, Blake S, Shrapnell K. Reaction to a diagnosis of breast cancer: relationship denial, delay and rates of psychological morbidity. *Cancer* 1984; 53:2008–2012.
29. Jackett TP CN. Development of a quantitative rating scale to assess denial. *J Psychosom Res* 1974; 18:93–100.
30. Cassileth BR, Zupkis RB, Sutton-Smith K, March V. Informed consent: Why are its goals imperfectly realized? *N Engl J Med* 1980; 302:896–900.
31. Cohen-Cole SA, Bird J. Interviewing the cardiac patient. In: Wenger N, editor. *A Practical Guide for Helping Patients Cope With Their Emotions*. New York: LeJacq Publishers, 1986, pp. 53–63.

32. Lazare A, Lipkin M, Putnam SM. The functions of the medical interview. In: Lipkin M, Putnam SM, Lazare A, editors. *The Medical Interview*. New York: Springer-Verlag, 2000.

33. Brody DS. The patient's role in clinical decision making. *Ann Intern Med* 1980; 93:718–722.

34. Quill TE. *A Midwife Through the Dying Proces: Stories of Healing and Hard Choices at the End of Life*. Baltimore: Johns Hopkins University Press, 1996.

7

Discussing Palliative Care with Patients

Palliative care focuses on relieving pain and other physical symptoms, enhancing psychosocial supports, and allowing patients and families to achieve meaningful resolution to their lives together. If suffering eventually increases out of proportion to prognosis, some patients choose palliation as the paramount goal of care. However, too many are never offered palliative care as a possibility, nor are they adequately informed when they are likely to be approaching the end of their lives. In addition, palliative care is frequently presented as an alternative to usual medical care, rather than something that can enhance or supplement it. Palliative care is often equated with hospice referral, which is frequently postponed until the patient is at the very brink of death.[1] Patients and families may then be deprived not only of adequate symptom management[2] but also of a full opportunity to say good-bye to one another. Why are these discussions so difficult and confusing that even experienced physicians struggle through them?

Barriers to Discussing Palliative Care

We live in a youth-oriented, death-denying society. While not completely taboo, discussions about death are outside of the mainstream. By comparison, in the pre-antibiotic era death was an integral part of family life, often occurring in the home. The death of a child from infectious illness was commonplace, and living to the age of 70 or 80 was the exception rather than the rule. As medicine has become more powerful and effective, average life expectancy has increased dramatically. At the same time, caring for the seriously ill has moved out of the home and into medical institutions. Despite remarkable medical successes, death paradoxically has become more alien and frightening.[3] Children are more likely to be kept out of the hospital and away from the deathbed of even an elderly relative. The motivation is not so much to protect the patient or the child against communicable disease as to protect the child (and thereby the rest of the family) from the sadness and potential trauma associated with illness and death. Instead of being an inevitable part of the life cycle, death seems unnatural and even more ominous, often attributed to a medical failure rather than an inevitable part of the human condition.

Simultaneous with our cultural alienation from death has come a deification of medical technology. We protect our citizens by guaranteeing cardiopulmonary resuscitation at the end of life unless they explicitly refuse. This brutal and frequently futile medical assault has essentially replaced more profound human and religious rituals that might allow a more peaceful and dignified closure to a person's life. When surveyed, a high percentage of U.S. citizens profess belief in a higher power,[4] yet there is a surprising absence of pastoral presence in the care of the severely ill and the dying. Clergy, in their churches, temples, and mosques, are not regularly entering into practical discussions about the challenges of death and dying. Instead of bedside vigils guided by clergy from a patient's personal religious tradition, the end of a person's life today is more likely to be characterized by intravenous tubing, indwelling catheters, and cardiac monitors. Most physical contact is from nurses and aides administering treatments and monitoring the patient's metabolic condition. The family, if present, may be dressed in gowns, masks, and gloves, observing monitors more than interacting with the patient, intimidated by technology rather than participating in care.

When people get sick, there is a powerful, almost religious belief that the right specialist, armed with the power of advanced medical technology, will be able to fix almost anything. Of course, many diseases that were without exception fatal only a few years ago are cured today. Renee Fox has written eloquently about the confusion that exists within the minds of patients, families, and physicians. Are medical failures the result of the limits inherent in medicine or the limited knowledge and abilities of one's particular practitioners?[5] The information explosion within medicine has contributed to this uncertainty, as well as to the dominance of the specialist, who narrows his or her spectrum of inquiry so that the amount of available medical information to be mastered is more manageable. Thus, severely ill patients are collectively cared for by teams of specialists, with each member overseeing a narrow spectrum of the patient's illness. These teams often lack a primary physician who watches out for the patient's overall well-being and serves as a translator and communicator between the providers, the patient, and the family. Consideration of palliative care issues tends to be postponed until all of the specialists agree that there is "nothing left to do" in each of their capacities. As a result, these discussions are often too late to allow for the kind of resolution that might have been possible had someone been continuously attending to the patient's overall condition and prognosis. Opening up a palliative care discussion involves acknowledging the possibility that aggressive treatment may not heal the patient, and that death may be in the offing. Since no one wants to hear such bad news, even if it reflects the patient's clinical reality, it is not hard to understand why such conversations are avoided.

Medical intervention is inherently probabilistic and always entails risk. This is difficult to grasp when it is one's own life and well-being hanging in the balance. Even with a treatment that is 95% likely to be effective, an informed patient will need to know what happens in the other 5% of cases.[6] If a bad outcome happens to you, even if it is improbable statistically, it is 100% likely that you will have to deal with the consequences.

As death approaches, the possibility of experimental therapy frequently has to be considered as an option. Even with the odds of such treatment working at 1 in 100, if you are that one person for whom it is effective, for you its efficacy is 100%. Why not at least try it? Here the informed patient and family will need to learn what "working" means—is it cure, or is it suppression of the disease for additional weeks or months? To be fully informed, a patient will also have to explore what happens to the other 99 patients for whom treatment does not "work," as this represents by far the more likely outcome. If a treatment is relatively benign, and the patient's quality of life is reasonably good (by his or her own estimation), then a clinical trial of experimental therapy frequently makes sense. On the other hand, if a treatment is toxic or if the patient already carries a large burden of suffering, such treatment may only decrease the quality of the patient's last days—days that might have been spent in other ways. I am not suggesting that aggressive experimental therapy is always unreasonable, but instead that a decision to proceed with it should be made as a result of a fully informed discussion that includes palliative options. Since death is the most likely outcome in any event, palliative care should be part of a treatment plan that includes even the most aggressive experimental therapy. Yet palliative care discussions acknowledge that death is on the horizon, and therefore may be simultaneously avoided by patient, family, and physicians.

To make matters worse, these challenging, emotionally laden discussions are generally not well reimbursed by insurance plans, especially when compared to the payment associated with technically invasive care. Not only may it be difficult at times to decide who among the medical team should initiate this discussion, but it may be hard to achieve a consensus among specialists managing the case that the time is right for such discussions. This is why I recommend that all severely ill patients decide with their doctors which health care provider will oversee their care. The physician can be a translator for the patient and family, and a negotiator on the patient's behalf with all of the specialists and others on the team. The clinician should have enough expertise to fully participate in medical decision making, but also be trusted by the patient and family to tell the truth and struggle with them to make the best decisions possible, often under adverse circumstances. For some, this individual might be their primary care physician. For others, one of the specialists on the team in whom they have the most confidence might be chosen.

A liberating part of these conversations is the realization that one does not have to give up on aggressive treatment directed toward underlying disease in order to explore palliative care issues.[7] There is no reason why *all* severely ill persons who *might* die in the next six to 12 months shouldn't be given the best pain management possible as well as the opportunity to work on issues of life closure. In viewing palliative care as independent from giving up traditional medical care, we are suddenly free to have end-of-life discussions with all severely ill patients, whether they want to continue aggressive treatment or pursue a predominantly palliative approach. Moving the subject of discussion away from accepting that one *is* dying to considering that one *might* die makes these important discussions less threatening—and they may occur much more frequently as a result.

When Should Palliative Care Be Discussed?

Although there is no clear consensus about when palliative care should be discussed, I believe that it is an absolute requirement under the following circumstances[8] (see Table 7–1):

1. *Patients fear future suffering.* Many patients and family members have seen relatives and friends struggle in the process of dying, and want to be reassured that they will be helped if they find themselves in such circumstances. Most patients find comfort in the promise of hospice programs to address their pain and other symptoms should they arise in the future, and with such reassurance they will then be free to spend their energy on other matters. Therefore, such fears present an excellent opportunity to inform the patient about the potential of palliative care.
2. *Patients or family members ask about hospice.* Such questions may be a subtext for exploring specific fears about the future, or they may be a sign

TABLE 7–1. Clinical Indications for Discussing Palliative Care

Absolute Indications

Patients fear future suffering

Patients or family members ask about hospice

Patients are imminently dying

Patients talk about wanting to die

Severe suffering and a poor prognosis

Potential Indications with Severely Ill Patients

When discussing the patient's hopes and fears

When discussing prognosis

Would you be surprised if the patient died in the next 6 months?

that a patient wants to readdress the goals of treatment or some currently unaddressed form of suffering. Clearly understanding why the question has been raised can lead to an exploration of the underlying meaning of the inquiry—for example, whether the patient is seeking reassurance about the future or is ready for transition to a hospice program.

3. *Patients are imminently dying.* Unfortunately, this is frequently the first time when palliative care issues are discussed. Discussion is timely and essential when death approaches suddenly and unexpectedly, because it is an absolute necessity to make the most of the time that remains. More frequently, death comes over a period of weeks, months, or more, and discussion is delayed until the last minute. Nevertheless, there is still opportunity for pain and symptom relief in the final hours to days of a person's life, and families can still come together around the patient.

4. *Patients talk about wanting to die.*[9] Sometimes inquiries about assisted dying are really requests for a shift in emphasis from restorative treatment to comfort-oriented treatment. Thus, a patient receiving intensive chemotherapy who makes such a request may simply be asking to stop active treatment directed at controlling cancer and shift to a predominantly palliative approach in a hospice program. There are many other reasons a patient might make such an inquiry, such as inadequate pain management, a family or spiritual crisis, or the emergence of serious depression. The patient may also be genuinely ready to die. Chapter 9 presents a strategy for evaluating and responding when a patient is exploring a wish to die in earnest.

5. *Patients have severe suffering and a poor prognosis.*[8] This is perhaps the most challenging scenario, for there are no absolute markers. One strong signal is when members of the health care team feel more and more uncomfortable administering aggressive therapy, or avoid even walking into the patient's room because of evident but unacknowledged suffering. Some clinicians may feel vaguely ill upon seeing the patient, and others that they are torturing the patient as much as or more than treating them. A survey of medical residents found that they frequently went against their conscience in treating patients invasively while under-treating pain and other uncomfortable symptoms.[10] Such patients are plentiful in today's hospitals, where only the sickest of the sick are admitted, and where diseases are managed to the highest degree possible while symptoms are frequently under-palliated.[11]

Perhaps discussions about palliative care should become a routine part of the care plan for all severely ill patients, even those who have a reasonably good chance of recovery. This will allow all patients to be better prepared in case their treatment does not go well, and will let them know that they have a right to good pain and symptom management whether they get better or not. Such discussions might occur under the following circumstances:

1. *When discussing the patient's hopes and fears.* Most severely ill patients hope for the best and imagine the worst. Fortunately they will talk about these matters if prompted, and many patients' fears can be easily reassured. For example, a patient whose worst fear is not being allowed enough pain medication in the future (perhaps based on a real-life experience with a relative or friend) can easily be reassured about the physician's willingness to prescribe all the pain medicine that might be needed.
2. *When discussing prognosis.* When a patient's prognosis is uncertain, there is usually a significant chance of a bad outcome. Rather than depriving a patient of hope, exploring the possibility of a bad outcome can be helpful with respect to reassuring the patient about the potential efficacy of hospice under such circumstances. Furthermore, considering such questions as "What would be left undone if you were to die sooner rather than later?" gives a dual message that time *may be* short, and that the patient may want to consider focusing attention on the most personally important and meaningful activities possible. To some degree, we should all be asking such questions, though they take on an immediacy when one is faced with serious, potentially fatal illness.
3. *Would you be surprised if the patient died within the next six months?*[7] Predicting when a patient will die is no easy matter, even with the best data and statistical modeling.[12] If we were to discuss palliative care with

only those patients who are dying with a high level of certainty, the field would be restricted to only a few diseases with the most predictable terminal trajectories. On the other hand, if we used the question above as our criterion for palliative care, we would broaden the field to include those who might die in the next few months but who also might live for several years. What is gained by this approach? A much larger population of seriously ill patients have access to better pain and symptom management, and have the opportunity to consider matters of life closure. Since palliative treatment does not preclude aggressive treatment of the person's underlying disease, there is little lost and much to be gained.

How Can Physicians Begin to Discuss Palliative Care?

General communications skills are needed to improve discussions with patients about palliative care. Because there are few rigorous outcome studies of communication explicitly directed to palliative care, the suggestions offered in the following sections stem from clinical experience, and analogy to research on physician–patient communication from other contexts.[13] Two hypothetical case scenarios illustrate potential questions and answers.

Mr. A. was a 54 year-old businessman who had colon cancer that had spread to his liver despite two regimens of chemotherapy. He was hospitalized because of bruises, oozing from blood-drawing sites, and nosebleeds. The previous evening, he had tripped on his way to the bathroom, cutting his arm and causing extensive bruising around his eyes. His chronic pain from widespread cancer was adequately controlled with around-the-clock long-acting morphine.

PHYSICIAN: *What is your understanding of where things stand now with your illness?*
MR. A.: *I know that the cancer is growing in my liver and that things don't look good.*
PHYSICIAN: *Yes, I wish that the liver lesions had gotten smaller.* (Pause.) *Tell me what is most important to you now.*
MR. A.: *I want to spend as much time as possible at home with my family.*
PHYSICIAN: *How is your family coping with all of this?*
MR. A.: (starts crying) *My daughter is afraid to be with me because of all the bruises and the black eyes.*

It is easy to imagine several ineffective ways that a physician might have responded in this conversation. The physician might not have checked the patient's understanding of his prognosis or inquired about his concerns, but instead talked about technical aspects of care, such as results of a blood count or clotting studies. When the patient said "things don't look good," the physician might have exhorted him not to lose hope and directed the discussion to experimental chemotherapy. When the patient began to cry, the physician might have squelched the discussion by turning the conversation to how adjusting medications might resolve the bleeding that frightened his daughter. Rather than prematurely trying to reassure the patient, or responding at a purely medical level, this physician continued to empathically explore Mr. A.'s experience.

PHYSICIAN: *What would you like to say to her when she is afraid?*

MR. A.: *(still crying) I want her to know that it is still me and that I love her more than she can ever know.*

PHYSICIAN: *You love her so much, it must feel terrible to think about leaving her.* (Pause.) *How can your time with your daughter be as meaningful as possible?*

The same simple interviewing techniques that physicians are trained to use in everyday clinical encounters can facilitate discussions in palliative care. These techniques include exploring the patient's perception of illness and prognosis, initiating discussion using open-ended questions, and then asking follow-up questions that incorporate the patient's own words.

In this interview, the physician first elicits the patient's concerns, goals, and values rather than discussing specific clinical decisions. After Mr. A.'s concerns and general goals are clarified, specific decisions, such as opting for a do-not-resuscitate order, may be easier to make. In contrast, many physicians begin by discussing specific management decisions and talk about palliative care only after a decision has been made to limit life-prolonging intervention.[14]

Open-ended questions generally are useful in eliciting patient concerns and emotions.[13] Table 7–2 lists potentially useful open-ended questions about

TABLE 7–2. Potentially Useful Open-Ended Questions about End-of-Life Care

---

"What concerns you most about your illness?"

"How is treatment going for you and your family?"

"As you think about your illness, what is the best and the worst that might happen?"

"What has been most difficult about this illness for you?"

"What are your hopes (your expectations, your fears) for the future?"

"As you think about the future, what is most important to you (what matters the most to you)?"

---

end-of-life care. These questions usually elicit an expansive answer and cannot be answered with a simple "yes" or "no." However, they focus attention on a particular domain of care and may direct attention to frequently avoided, emotionally significant issues.

The patient's own language can then guide the physician's follow-up responses and questions. Using Mr. A.'s own words communicates that he is being carefully listened to and that his perspective is important. Patients who sense that they are understood may feel more comfortable in disclosing additional concerns and emotions. Subsequent comments by the physician that build on the patient's responses can help in acknowledging the patient's emotions, exploring their meaning, and encouraging the patient to say more about difficult topics.[15,16] Some physicians may fear that focusing attention on emotions may scare the patient and family or create feelings of hopelessness and despair that they are powerless to alleviate. However, patients and families have these emotional responses whether or not the physician chooses to probe them. At a minimum, once these emotions are discussed openly, the patient and family are no longer alone with them. Furthermore, fear, anxiety, and depression may be amenable to simple interventions once they are fully understood. Rather than avoiding Mr. A.'s grief regarding his daughter, the physician can explore how he might talk to her about his illness and death.

PHYSICIAN: (addressing Mrs. A.) *I would like to know if you have any additional concerns.*

MRS. A.: *I am scared that he will bleed uncontrollably at home, and I won't know what to do. I would call 911 if this happens. At least they can help me.*

With the patient's consent, physicians can involve close family members in discussions about palliative care. Family members frequently raise additional issues, and their cooperation may be essential for some health care options. For example, most patients in hospice need a committed primary caregiver at home. Mrs. A.'s major fear is not her husband's death but rather whether she will be able to handle the final stages of his dying. Physicians may hesitate to ask about the patient's or family's concerns for fear of being asked to address an unsolvable problem. Indeed, uncontrollable bleeding can be difficult to palliate. However, understanding and attempting to address Mrs. A.'s concerns is an essential first step before plans are made for Mr. A. to return home.

PHYSICIAN (to Mrs. A.): *Yes, bleeding can be frightening, particularly if you're at home with your daughter. Are there other things that are frightening or too much to handle?*

MRS. A.: *I know Jim wants to be home, and I want that too. But sometimes it feels like I'm in too far over my head.*

After Mrs. A.'s concerns are fully elucidated, the physician can then explain how hospice provides support for care at home, including 24-hour access by telephone, home visits on short notice for such events as major bleeding, and admission to an inpatient palliative care unit if needed.[17]

Physicians sometimes shy away from terms like *hospice* or *palliative care* because they imply that death is imminent.[18] However, euphemisms, such as *supportive care*, *comfort care*, and *comprehensive care*, may be ambiguous or misleading. Whatever language is used, physicians should make sure a common understanding of the term's meanings exists. It can be useful to discuss or provide specific examples of the elements of palliative care, such as pain management and family support, without labeling them palliative or terminal care.

During these emotionally intense encounters, physicians must remember to ask directly about the patient's symptoms. This information is necessary to provide relief. A "review of systems" of common problems for dying patients should include pain, fatigue, shortness of breath, and symptoms specific to the site of the patient's illness. If pain is present, the physician should ask the patient to quantify it on a numeric scale.[19] Screening for depression is essential, because depression is common and often overlooked.[20] The simple question *"Are you depressed?"* may be a useful screening tool.[21]

Stoic patients may deny physical or psychosocial distress. In such circumstances, the physician can gather information about the patient's needs indirectly by asking such questions as *"How is your wife [daughter, son, etc.] dealing with your illness?"* The physician can pose follow-up questions based on the patient's responses, allowing the patient to explore the impact of his or her illness on family members. Another approach is to ask, *"Have any family members or friends had a similar illness?"* If the patient answers in the affirmative, the physician might ask what symptoms or concerns they experienced. Some patients find that they can express fears and concerns "once removed" —that is, through the experiences of a family member or friend.

Most experts believe that attention to spiritual, existential, and religious issues is a crucial component of palliative care.[22] The physician's role in checking these domains for conflict or unfinished business is essential. On the other hand, the physician's responsibility for following through with these discussions is more controversial, because physicians vary in their interest, comfort, and skills in these areas. Given the opportunity, a patient may choose to talk to a pastor, priest, rabbi, or other spiritual adviser with whom he or she has an existing relationship and who may be best suited to help the patient come to terms with mortality and find meaning in the final stage of life. Physicians can help arrange contact with an appropriate religious or spiritual adviser: *"These are important issues. I'd be glad to arrange for a pastor [priest, rabbi, chaplain or cleric] to meet with you."* Even if physicians do not personally discuss these

TABLE 7–3. Potentially Useful Questions about Spiritual and Existential Issues

"Is faith (religion, spirituality) important to you?"

"Would you like to explore religious matters with someone?"

"What do you still want to accomplish during your life?"

"What thoughts have you had about why you got this illness at this time?"

"What might be left undone if you were to die today?"

"What is your understanding of what happens after you die?"

"Given that your time is limited, what legacy do you want to leave your family?"

"What do you want your children and grandchildren to remember about you?"

issues in depth with their patients, they can validate the importance of such topics and encourage the patient to continue to explore them.

Patients who lack formal religious affiliation, have lost faith, are alienated from their religion, or are atheist or agnostic may prefer to discuss spiritual and existential issues with their physicians. In one patient poll, 39% of respondents considered it very important to have a physician who was spiritually attuned to them.[23] Whatever their own views, physicians or other members of the health care team should screen for unaddressed spiritual and existential concerns. Table 7–3 suggests questions that may help to initiate such discussions.

How Can Physicians Respond to Difficult Patient Statements and Questions?

Not surprisingly, a patient's answers to open-ended questions can be disturbing or difficult to respond to. Suppose that Mr. A. said the most important thing for him was to be alive for his daughter's birthday, almost a year away. If the physician believes that Mr. A. has a 90% chance of dying within six months, how might he respond? He might say directly, *"I wish I could tell you that you will be here for your daughter's next birthday. It is possible, but unfortunately the odds aren't with you. (Pause.) If it doesn't work out that you can be there, are there things that you should consider doing now?"* An interpretative comment (*"It must be frightening to think about not being with her."*) is riskier because it goes beyond the patient's statement; however, it may also validate the patient's underlying emotion and encourage further discussion. As an alternative, the physician might say, *"I know that you're trying very hard to keep your hopes up. Are you sometimes afraid that you won't be there for your family?"* This response aligns the physician with the patient's wish without reinforcing unrealistic plans. Later, the physician might say, *"What would you want to say to your daughter on her birthday?"* By returning to Mr. A.'s original wish about his daughter's birthday, this question might lead to a discussion of making a videotaped message for his daughter.

Discussions about palliative care may uncover problems without solutions. Some patients no longer find meaning in life or fear punishment in the after-life; some families are overwhelmed or have long-standing conflicts that defy solution. When patients reveal such concerns, physicians may feel that their probing has made the situation worse. In these difficult situations, physicians should keep in mind several points: First, uncovering painful emotions does seem to increase short-term suffering. In the longer term, however, exploring such difficult issues may lessen feelings of aloneness and raise opportunities to find comfort and resolution. Second, the physician's feelings are often an impor-tant clue to how the patient is feeling. For example, if the physician feels over-whelmed, frustrated, discouraged, or angry, the patient may well have similar feelings. Sharing such feelings may lessen isolation and lead to an experience of connectedness for both patient and physician.[24] Third, physicians can clarify their own role and self-expectations. Physicians do not need to fix all identified problems. Being a "fellow traveler" who understands and listens carefully to insoluble problems often is therapeutic; patients no longer feel alone with their problems if they believe that their concerns have been heard. Physicians should recall that the term *compassion* comes from the Latin words for "feel with" or "suffer with". Statements such as "I wish that medicine had better answers" may show alliance with the patient's hopes and be more soothing than we suspect. Finally, physicians do not have sole responsibility for responding to the patient's suffering; they can call on nurses, social workers, chaplains, psycholo-gists, and psychiatrists for help.[17]

Patients and families frequently have hard questions that they may or may not ask the physician or nurse (see Table 7–4). The more trust in the medical relationship, the more likely that these questions will surface. This can be facil-itated by giving the patient and family permission to ask any question they might have. Although there is no formula for answering these questions, the following are ideas about which approach might best address their underlying meaning and importance.

1. *"How long do I have?"* Most experts agree that a rigid time limit should not be given in response to this query, in part because of medicine's inherent prognostic uncertainty. Many patients who outlive their initial prognosis will remember with pride and anger a doctor who inaccurately told them that they had "six months to live". Nevertheless, if the patient is very likely to die in three to six months, he or she may need to know that to do appropriate planning. When asked, I generally try to give the patient ballpark averages, but always include the possibility of an excep-tion (in either direction.) *"The usual person with your condition will live*

TABLE 7–4. Some Difficult Questions

"How long do I have?"

"What would you do in my shoes?"

"Should I try or experimental (or complementary) therapy?"

"Should I go to a 'medical mecca' for treatment or a second opinion?"

"Will you work with me all the way through to my death, no matter what happens?"

"If my suffering gets really bad, will you help me die?"

three to six months, but there are always people who beat the odds and live a lot longer, and a few who live shorter. I hope you will be in the group that outlives this prognosis, but unfortunately we can't count on it, so we'd better prepare for all possibilities."

2. *"What would you do in my shoes?"* Although I am a staunch advocate of patient choice and autonomy, I believe that we have an obligation to try to answer such questions, putting ourselves in the patient's shoes and respecting his or her values as much as possible. The answer should always be qualified—for example, "I can't be sure what I would actually do," or "My answer will be influenced to some degree by my own values, which may be different from yours." Yet most patients want us to use both our professional judgment and our personal experience to come up with a recommendation.[25] The final choice is ultimately the patient's, but he or she may benefit from our considered opinion.

3. *"Should I try experimental (or complementary) therapy?"* Responses to questions about experimental therapy depend in part on a patient's underlying condition, personal values, and degree of suffering, and on the particular experimental therapy's toxicity, invasiveness, and likelihood of working. It is important to clarify whether the goal of treatment is cure or extension of life for a few months, so the patient can make a fully informed decision. There is no reason not to provide excellent palliative care even if aggressive experimental therapy is initiated, for such treatment is unlikely to cure most diseases, and death is likely to still be in the patient's near future. Similarly, some patients may want to pursue complementary or alternative treatments with which a physician may be unfamiliar. It is incumbent upon the physician to help the patient evaluate such treatments in terms of potential efficacy and meaning, as well as expense and toxicity. Noninvasive complementary practices can often enhance a palliative care treatment plan for patients

who want to explore what non-allopathic traditions have to offer at this stage of life.

4. *"Should I go to a 'medical mecca' for treatment or for a second opinion?"* Part of the deification of medical technology and of the medical expert is the pilgrimage to a highly specialized medical center for potential treatment. Second opinions from highly specialized physicians can be worthwhile, especially for patients with rare conditions. However, such institutions tend to err on the aggressive side of treatment, and often do not fully explore the downside of such treatments—for example, added suffering and spending more of one's last days in medical institutions. A second opinion does not obligate the patient to accept recommended treatment, but it can be valuable in validating options and making sure that no possibilities have remained unexplored.

5. *"Will you work with me all the way through to my death, no matter what happens?"* This is a request for partnership and for nonabandonment[26] through the dying process. Those patients and families who have this commitment from their physicians face the end of life less afraid, particularly if their fears have been explored and addressed. The commitment is open-ended, since the clinician does not exactly know what will be asked for or needed. Yet this is the uncertainty that patients and families are confronted with, and those with a committed medical partner are fortunate.

6. *"If my suffering gets really bad, will you help me die?"* This question may seem threatening to many physicians. Chapter 9 presents an approach to answering it. After exploring the patient's fears and concerns, the first place to go in search of a response is standard palliative care, which emphasizes a commitment to aggressive pain and symptom management. Many good palliative care doctors, even those who are adamantly opposed to physician-assisted suicide, answer this question in the affirmative. They commit to aggressive palliative care, including unlimited access to pain medication up to and including terminal sedation if needed.[27] Potential last-resort methods are explored in Chapter 12. The reassurance this commitment provides can be invaluable to those who fear a bad death or may have witnessed one in their own family.

How Can Physicians Discuss Palliative Care While Disease-Remitting Treatments Are Continued?

Mrs. D. was an 82 year-old woman with diabetes mellitus, renal insufficiency, coronary artery disease, and congestive heart failure. Her two daughters lived in the same building, and did her housework and shopping. Mrs. D. was hospitalized for the third time in two months because of angina and an exacerbation of congestive heart failure. The following conversation occured at a family meeting:

PHYSICIAN: *Mrs. D., what concerns you most about your condition?*

MRS. D.: *I hate feeling that I can't breathe. What's going to happen if my breathing gets worse? I would rather be dead than go to a nursing home, but I also feel that I'm a burden on my daughters. I used to be so independent!*

MRS. D.'S DAUGHTER: *Mom, you are not a burden! We will do whatever it takes to keep you out of a nursing home.*

Like Mrs. D.'s daughter, the physician might have tried to reassure her immediately. The physician could have attempted this in several ways. He could have focused exclusively on the biological aspects of care—for example, discussing how angioplasty might improve circulation to her heart so that she would not need to depend on her daughter. As an alternative, the physician could have said that her daughters obviously loved her deeply and were glad to help her. Premature reassurance, although usually well-intentioned, often forecloses exploration of inherently challenging dimensions of the patient's illness. Instead of limiting discussion, the physician began to explore the patient's concerns by building on her statements:

PHYSICIAN: *In what ways do you feel like a burden?*

MRS. D.: *I am terrified of being alone when my daughters are at work. What if something happens and I suddenly can't breathe? My daughters have to work, and they can't spend their whole lives caring for me. Yet I don't want to go to a nursing home.*

PHYSICIAN: *You sound very distressed about the possibility of a nursing home. What is the worst part of that for you?*

When this line of inquiry is complete, the physician might explore the patient's other main fear of being unable to breathe as her condition deteriorates:

PHYSICIAN: *What frightens you the most about your breathing?*

MRS. D.: *The feeling of suffocation is so frightening. I am not at all afraid of death, but I am terrified of drowning along the way. I am not sure how I would handle it if I become severely short of breath!*

By encouraging Mrs. D. to say more about her concerns, the physician begins to hear about the core issues and fears with which she is struggling. To further probe her concerns, the physician uses Mrs. D.'s own words about being a burden or going to a nursing home or suffocating. Naturally, physicians want to reassure patients. However, reassurance may deter patients from disclosing their concerns and emotions in enough detail that they can be understood.[28] In addition, offering reassurance before fully understanding patients' concerns may paradoxically increase their worry about the future. Eliciting and openly discussing Mrs. D.'s fears enabled her physician to develop a comprehensive, individualized plan to address her problems. Although Mrs. D. did not want major surgery, she eventually agreed to angioplasty in hopes of improving her angina and congestive heart failure, which would allow her to become more active and independent. In addition, the family and social worker eventually looked into a geriatric day care program so that Mrs. D. would not be alone as much during the day and her daughters could continue to work.

Because Mrs. D. was frightened about feeling short of breath, the physician began discussing how severe shortness of breath might be approached in the future. Morphine is one of the best symptom-relieving measures for severe shortness of breath; the physician eventually suggested having the daughters learn to administer it to Mrs. D. at home if needed.

MRS. D.'S DAUGHTER: *Wait, you're not giving up on her, are you?*

PHYSICIAN: *Absolutely not! Morphine is one of the most effective medicines we have to relieve shortness of breath. I will explain more in a minute. But first can you tell me what you mean by "giving up"?*

The physician's initial response to the daughter is an unqualified expression of nonabandonment[26] and a clarification of the role of morphine in palliating shortness of breath. He follows this with a focused inquiry to clarify the daughter's perception of "giving up." Later, the physician can explore the daughter's concern about the use of morphine by asking, "*What have you heard about morphine to relieve shortness of breath or pain?*" Common misconceptions are that opioids are dangerous, cause addiction, shorten life, and are used only as a last resort. In fact, they are relatively safe, rarely if ever cause addiction or respiratory depression in the terminally ill, and are mainstays of therapy for shortness of breath as well as for pain.[29] The physician can explain that morphine may relieve severe shortness of breath at home if nitroglycerin and oxygen are ineffective. He can also explain that paramedics often use morphine for patients with severe heart failure. Later the physician can discuss decisions about hospice, resuscitation, and intubation.[30] It would also be useful to check with Mrs. D. and her daughters about whether the suggested plan addresses their concerns.

Objections to This Approach

Some physicians may object to this approach of using open-ended questions, following up on the patient's answers by asking questions using the patient's own words, and adding empathic comments where appropriate. They may interpret the method as leaving the physician's own views out of the exchange. However, once this "patient-centered" inquiry is completed, physicians should not be afraid to draw on their clinical experience to give patients recommendations for medical care.[25] This is particularly important when patients ask physicians directly what they would do, in the same situation, for themselves or for a loved one. In my opinion, this is part of what most patients are asking for from their physicians. Final decisions about how to proceed belong to the patient, but patients should not be deprived of the physician's professional as well as personal thoughts on the subject.

Some physicians go further in sharing with patients thoughts on death and spirituality or anecdotes about good deaths from their own experience. Other physicians choose not to share their personal views of a good death, instead concentrating as much as possible on the patient's values, spirituality, and experience. These physicians believe that the focus should remain as much as possible on the patient, and strive to avoid imposing their own views. Moreover, active listening and empathic communication may be more likely than self-disclosure to result in patient disclosures that facilitate a personal connection.[24] Regardless of their willingness to share with patients their own views on dying, physicians can try to comfort patients by listening closely to their concerns and accurately identifying their feelings.

In a multicultural society, a physician's patients may have widely varying attitudes toward discussions of death. In some cultures there is widespread belief that discussion of death hastens its occurrence,[30,31] so advance planning about end-of-life care may be inappropriate for a patient from one of these cultures. Usually, however, it is still possible to talk sensitively about the alleviation of suffering, concerns about the future, or how serious illness is managed and discussed in the patient's culture. And because people within every culture vary, each patient and family needs to be approached as a unique member of that culture. The more the clinician starts with an open-ended inquiry and uses the patient's own language to build follow–up questions, the more likely he or she can keep the inquiry focused on the individual patient. The approaches recommended earlier in this chapter encourage the physician to listen carefully and allow the patient's concerns to drive the discussion, ensuring respect for each patient's values and culture.

Concluding Thoughts

Palliative care is important to consider throughout the course of serious chronic illness. Interviewing techniques, such as asking open-ended questions about end-of-life issues, building on and exploring patient responses, and addressing associated emotions, can help initiate difficult discussions about palliative care. In addition to addressing physical suffering, physicians can extend their care by acknowledging and exploring psychosocial, existential, or spiritual suffering. As patients struggle to find resolution in their lives, active listening and empathy have therapeutic value in and of themselves.

- *Note*: Many of the ideas in the sections titled "How can physicians begin to discuss palliative care?", "How can physicians discuss palliative care while disease-remitting treatments are continued?", and Tables 7–2 and 7–3 were originally presented in an article I coauthored with Bernie Lo and James Tulsky titled "Discussing palliative care," *Annals of Internal Medicine* 1999; 130:744–749, as part of the ACP/ASIM End-of-Life Consensus Panel. I gratefully acknowledge their generosity in letting me use that material, and I am solely responsible for the additional sections and editing.

References

1. Christakis NA. Timing of referral of terminally ill patients to an outpatient hospice. *J Gen Intern Med* 1994; 9:314–320.
2. *Approaching Death: Improving Care at the End of Life*. Washington, DC: National Academy Press, 1997.
3. Aries P. *The Hour of Our Death*. New York: Oxford University Press, 1991.
4. Grey A. The spiritual component of palliative care. *Palliat Med* 1994; 8:215–221.
5. Fox R. *Experiment Perilous: Physicians and Patients Facing the Unknown*. Glencoe, Ill: Free Press, 1959.
6. Tversky A, Kahneman D. The framing of decisions and the psychology of choice. *Science* 1982; 211:453–458.
7. Lynn J. Caring at the end of our lives. *N Engl J Med* 1996; 335:201–202.
8. Quill TE. Initiating end-of-life discussions with severely ill patients: Addressing the "elephant in the room." *JAMA* 2000; 284:2502–2507.
9. Quill TE. Doctor, I want to die. Will you help me? *JAMA* 1993; 270:870–873.
10. Solomon MZ, O'Donnell L, Jennings B, Guilfoy V, Wolf SM, Nolan K, et al. Decisions near the end of life: Professional views on life-sustaining treatments. *Am J Public Health* 1993; 83:14–23.
11. The SUPPORT Principal Investigators. A controlled trial to improve care for seriously ill hospitalized patients. The study to understand prognoses and preferences for outcomes and risks of treatment (SUPPORT). *JAMA* 1995; 274:1591–1598.
12. Lynn J, Harrell F Jr, Cohn F, Wagner D, Connors AF Jr. Prognoses of seriously ill hospitalized patients on the days before death: implications for patient care and public policy. *New Horizons* 1997; 5(1):56–61.
13. Lazare A, Lipkin M, Putnam SM. The functions of the medical interview. In: Lipkin M, Putnam SM, Lazare A, editors. *The Medical Interview*. New York: Springer-Verlag, 2000.
14. Tulsky J, Chesney MA, Lo B. How do medical residents discuss resuscitation with patients? *J Gen Intern Med* 1995; 10:436–442.

15. Buckman R, Kason Y. *How to Break Bad News: A Guide for Health Care Professionals.* Baltimore: The Johns Hopkins University Press, 1992.
16. Suchman AL, Markakis K, Beckman HB, Frankel R. A model of empathic communication in the medical interview. *JAMA* 1997; 277:678–682.
17. Doyle D, Hanks GW, MacDonald N. *Oxford Textbook of Palliative Medicine*, 2nd ed. New York: Oxford University Press, 1998.
18. Billings JA. What is palliative care? *J Palliat Care* 1998; 1:73–81.
19. Foley KM. The treatment of cancer pain. *N Engl J Med* 1989; 313:84–95.
20. Block SD. Assessing and managing depression in the terminally ill patient. ACP-ASIM End-of-Life Care Consensus Panel. *Ann Intern Med* 2000; 132:209–218.
21. Chochinov HM, Wilson KG, Enns M, Lander S. "Are you depressed?" Screening for depression in the terminally ill. *Am J Psychiatry* 1997; 154:674–676.
22. Kirschling JM, Pittman JF. Measurement of spiritual well-being: a hospice caregiver sample. *Hospice Journal* 1989; 5:1–11.
23. Monroe B. Social work aspects of palliative care. In: Doyle D, Hanks GW, MacDonald N, editors. *Oxford Textbook of Palliative Medicine.* Oxford: Oxford University Press, 1998:867–882.
24. Matthews DA, Suchman AL, Branch WT Jr. Making "connexions": Enhancing the therapeutic potential of patient-clinician relationships. *Ann Intern Med* 1993; 118:973–977.
25. Quill TE, Brody H. Physician recommendations and patient autonomy: Finding a balance between physician power and patient choice. *Ann Intern Med* 1996; 125:763–769.
26. Quill TE, Cassel CK. Nonabandonment: A central obligation for physicians. *Ann Intern Med* 1995; 122:368–374.
27. Byock IR. When suffering persists . . . *J Palliat Care* 1994; 10:8–13.
28. Faulkner A, Maguire P. *Talking to Cancer Patients and Their Relatives.* New York: Oxford University Press, 1994.
29. Graber MA, Levy BI, Weir RF, Oppliger RA. Patients' views about physician participation in assisted suicide and euthanasia. *J Gen Intern Med* 1996; 11:71–76.
30. Tulsky J, Fischer GS, Rose MR, Arnold RM. Opening the black box: How do physicians communicate about advance directives? *Ann Intern Med* 1998; 129:441–449.
31. Blackhall LJ, Murphy ST, Frank G, Michel V, Azan S. Ethnicity and attitudes toward patient autonomy. *JAMA* 1995; 274:820–825.

8

Palliative Care for Patients with Severe Dementia: A Consensus-Based Approach to Decision Making

As we grow older the world becomes stranger, the pattern more
complicated of dead and living.
                                        —T. S. Eliot, "East Coker"

Mrs. B. was a 73 year-old woman with severe Alzheimer's disease. She
was a retired schoolteacher with a husband and daughter. For the previous
three years, she had lived in a nursing home and required assistance with
all of her basic activities of daily living. Mr. B. visited her daily and fed her
lunch. In the past several weeks, she had taken longer to finish small
portions of food. At times, she coughed while being fed. One morning
after breakfast, Mrs. B. developed agitation, a cough, shortness of breath,
and a temperature of 100.3 degrees.

Palliative care is designed to relieve a patient's suffering in order to maximize dignity and quality of life.[1] Respect for a patient's autonomous choices
is a foundation of Western bioethics, but a patient with severe dementia can

An earlier version of this chapter was coauthored with Jason Karlawish and Diane Meier, and
was published in the *Annals of Internal Medicine* 1999; 130:835–840 as part of the American
College of Physicians–American Society of Internal Medicine (ACP/ASIM) End-of-Life Care
Consensus Panel. I am responsible for all additions and subsequent editing.

119

no longer decide whether to receive predominantly palliative care or to continue potentially life-prolonging therapy. Although severe Alzheimer's diease is used in this chapter as an example, the principles illustrated can be generalized to other mentally incapacitated adults. Other people, such as family members and caregivers, must make medical decisions for the patient. The goals and values of these decision makers may conflict with those of each other and with those of the patient, who now lacks the capacity to participate in the decision. Conflicts are especially likely in decision making about two common clinical problems that result from neurologically based swallowing difficulties: malnutrition and pneumonia. These problems engage deep values about feeding, starvation, and the meaning of care.[2] Furthermore, a patient's residence in a nursing home introduces additional problems related to regulations governing the management of a patient's weight loss and nutrition.[3] How can a busy clinician address these problems in a manner that achieves consensus among decision makers? This case study illustrates an approach to developing palliative care plans for severely ill patients who cannot speak for themselves.

At a meeting with Mr. B. and his daughter, the physician explains that aspiration pneumonia is a common problem in severe stages of dementia caused by an irreversible and progressive loss of the ability to chew and swallow food. Mr. B. agrees that his wife has had trouble eating, and he describes how on some days she eats very little of even her favorite foods.

To prompt the family to tell more about their perception of how Mrs. B. has changed, the physician asks, "I know that Mrs. B. was diagnosed with Alzheimer's over seven years ago, but I have known her only for the last few months. Can you tell me how she seems to you now, and how things have changed compared to when she was first admitted?"

The family's story begins with a summer vacation cut short seven years ago when Mrs. B. fell and was hospitalized for 10 days. She never fully recovered, and she experienced a progressive loss of function over the ensuing years. The physician listened carefully to the family's story, and responded to the emotions of sadness and anger that were associated with relentless losses that accompanied Mrs. B.'s decline.

After fully hearing about the family's experience, the physician responded by saying, "I think I have a better understanding about how things have changed over the past few years. It sounds like both you and she have done the best you could through a difficult situation. You know that Mrs. B. has an incurable, progressive, and ultimately fatal disease. I can't say for sure when she'll die of her Alzheimer's disease, but given its severity, we shouldn't be surprised when she does. Even if she does recover from this bout of pneumonia, she will not recover her swallowing function. Recognizing this, we ought to care for her in a way that makes us confident that, after she's gone, we can say she was treated with dignity and respect.

"I use two principles to help think through the decisions we face. First, consider your understanding of what Mrs. B. would want if she could tell us. Second, let's try to balance the burdens and benefits of each option in terms of its ability to relieve her suffering and maximize her dignity and the quality of her remaining life."

This narrative initiates an emotional and meaningful dialogue that should lead to a consensus about the best way to care for Mrs. B. given her clinical circumstances. This consensus-based approach is distinct from a discussion in which individuals simply share their opinions but there is no genuine attempt to reconcile their differences. The process and pitfalls of consensus building will vary depending on the patient's clinical condition, family dynamics, and the level of preexisting trust or conflict in the physician–patient–family relation ship. Nevertheless, a physician can guide this dialogue by using the goals and steps that are outlined in Tables 8–1 and 8–2 and discussed below.

A physician's first step is to identify potential decision makers. In Mrs. B.'s case, had she completed an advance directive that included a durable power of attorney for health care, that person would be her main representative in decision making. However, most patients in nursing homes do not have advance directives.[4] Even when they do, other family members, caregivers with special knowledge about the patient, and other members of the health care team can greatly assist the designated surrogate in decision making.[5-7] If a patient does

TABLE 8–1. The Core Principles with Which to Plan Palliative Care for Patients Who Lack Decision-Making Capacity

Structure decision making as a consensus-building process grounded in dialogue among proxy, other close family members, physician, and immediate caregivers.

The goal is to achieve consensus about:
- diagnosis and prognosis
- benefits and burdens of different treatment options
- meaning of emotionally charged terms (e.g. starvation, suffering, quality of life, feeding, and dying)

Decisions should be based on:
- patient's preferences
- balance of the burdens and benefits

Palliative care should be offered whether life-prolonging measures are initiated or the patient is treated with comfort measures only.

TABLE 8–2. Steps to Providing Palliative Care to Patients Who Lack Decision-Making Capacity

STEP	REPRESENTATIVE QUOTE TO ACHIEVE STEP
1. Identify the main participants in the decision making.	*"We need to make some decisions about the care of your wife. Is everyone here who could help us think through what we should do?"*
2. Allow the participants to narrate how the patient has come to this stage of illness (or, in cases where the physician has had an extended relationship with the patient and family).	*"Can you tell me how things have changed; how things have gone for each of you?" [or, "I know I've been caring for your wife for many years, but it helps me if you can tell me how she has changed, and how things have gone for each of you."]*
3. Teach the decision makers about the expected clinical course of the patient's disease.	*"Your wife has an incurable, progressive, and ultimately fatal disease. I can't say for sure when she will die from Alzheimer's disease, but given its severity, we shouldn't be surprised when she does."*
4. Advocate for the patient's quality of life and dignity.	*"We ought to take care of her in a way that makes us confident that after she is gone, we can say she was treated with dignity and respect."*
5. Provide guidance on the basis of existing data and clinical experience.	*"For patients like Mrs. B., feeding with a tube does not significantly reduce the risk of pneumonia. On the basis of my experience, a speech therapist can give us some useful hints on ways to feed her that will allow her to continue to eat by mouth."*

not have an advance directive, the physician can turn to close family members and others who know the patient well with the assurance that the family's standing to serve as surrogate decision makers is established by both case and statutory law.[8] Except in cases in which the patient has no family or has a family that appears unable to represent the patient's best interests, the physician is under no moral or legal authority to seek a guardian.[8-10]

After identifying the decision makers and clarifying Mrs. B.'s diagnosis, the physician encouraged them to describe the course of Mrs. B.'s dementia by asking how she has changed. The purpose of this dialogue was to achieve a consensus among the decision makers about the patient's current disease state, prognosis, quality of life, and previously stated values.[6] This sharing of narratives may expose important differences in beliefs and understandings in any of these domains, which must be reconciled before consensus-based decision making can proceed. The more the physician understands these various perceptions, the more likely he or she will be able to develop a plan that will respect Mrs. B. as a person. Even when a physician has a long-term relationship with a family and patient, this step in consensus building should not be skipped. Research showing that physicians often inadequately understand their patients' preferences for health care supports this assertion.[11–14]

The next step in consensus building is to begin a dialogue about prognosis and about a potential role of palliative care. This was done with the phrase that ended *"Mrs. B. has an incurable, progressive, and ultimately fatal disease."* Although this physician believes strongly in a palliative approach that includes pain and symptom management and avoids invasive treatments for patients with severe Alzheimer's disease, he must respect that others may value an approach in which available medical technology is used to prolong life. Before a consensus about what might be included in a palliative approach for a particular patient is possible, the physician must learn what *"treated with dignity and respect"* means to this family.

In Mrs. B.'s case, the physician guided the family on ethical standards for decision making. They were asked to: (1) consider what is known of the patient's wishes and preferences given her current condition (for example, referral to a living will or potentially relevant statements made when the patient was competent); and (2) balance the burdens and benefits of each option in terms of its ability to maximize Mrs. B.'s dignity and quality of life. Deciding how to care for Mrs. B. by using only a rigid understanding of her past preferences may fail to respect her present circumstances.[15] Achieving consensus about her current quality of life, although a subjective and personal process, incorporates the family's, physician's, and health care team's perceptions of her current circumstances into what is known about her past preferences and values.

Missing from these recommendations to the family is an exclusive appeal to futility as grounds for decision making. Futility refers to a claim that no desirable benefit can be achieved by potentially life-prolonging treatment.[16] Physicians frequently cite futility as their reason for terminating further treatment.[17] Although the concept of "medical futility" exists to communicate extremely poor prognosis, it can also inadvertently convey an unequivocal, unilateral, and negative judgment about a patient's quality of life without leading to an explicit discussion of these issues from the differing perspectives of physicians and families. Furthermore, too frequently the term connotes that "nothing more can be done" for a patient, that further intervention would be meaningless, or that the patient's life is of no current value. Therefore, a physician who relies exclusively on futility as a reason to pursue palliative care can obscure an honest discussion of how people understand and value the patient's continued existence and of the range of possibilities for palliative and life-prolonging interventions.

Mr. B. and his daughter agree that Mrs. B. never expressed clear preferences about how she should be treated. The physician reassures them that they can still work on a plan. He outlines the options, including transfer to the hospital or staying at the nursing home with or without antibiotic therapy, and explains his view of their benefits and burdens. "A helpful way to think through these choices is to come to some consensus about her current quality of life, and then decide which options will maximize it."

In the ensuing discussion, Mrs. B.'s daughter and the physician state that they feel Mrs. B.'s quality of life is poor because she cannot communicate or move around. Her husband disagrees. "I know she still hears me and understands me. I can see it in her eyes when I bring her food from home." The daughter begins to cry and says that her mother would not want to live the way she is. Again, the husband disagrees. "You're not here every day! I am!" This common conflict challenges the consensus-building process.

The physician looks for common ground by asking them: "If she gets worse, if she can't recognize you or starts to suffer more, do we all agree that we should focus purely on her comfort and that even antibiotics would be too invasive?" The husband starts to cry and is comforted by the daughter. They both nod in agreement.

The physician then proposes a compromise plan. "Mr. B., your visits are important. I recommend that we keep her here at the nursing home where you can visit her as much as possible. We can simultaneously provide antibiotics and try our best to keep her comfortable. If she deteriorates, our focus can shift exclusively to relieving her symptoms and minimizing her immediate suffering. I strongly recommend against providing cardiopulmonary resuscitation should she have a cardiac arrest, since I don't think it would work. It would only add to her suffering."

The family agrees that the plan strikes a proper balance between benefits and burdens, giving her a chance of recovery without subjecting her to a foreign environment or overly harsh treatments.

This decision-making process exposed two common features of caring for patients with severe dementia. First, clear information about the patient's wishes is typically unavailable. Second, decision makers often have differing assessments of the patient's preferences and quality of life.[18] In this case, the daughter and the physician thought that Mrs. B. had a poor quality of life and were concerned that hospitalization and even antibiotics might further decrease her quality of life. The husband disagreed. They all were genuinely trying to act in Mrs. B.'s best interests without clear information about her preferences. They achieved compromise with the decision to give Mrs. B. a therapeutic trial of antibiotics at the nursing home.

Dialogue is essential to achieve consensus on a course of action that is responsive to both past and present patient realities, as well as to the concerns and priorities of the family.[5–7,19] The goal of dialogue is not to provoke conflict but to clarify common ground and differences and lead to better appreciation of the meaning of the decision for the patient and her family.[6,20] This approach to decision making is grounded in narrative theory that unifies the clinical and moral dimensions of medicine.[9,21,22] Clinical medicine is grounded in a series of stories told and interpreted from a variety of perspectives. The physician usually interprets these stories, using the science of clinical medicine to develop a diagnostic and therapeutic plan. These same stories can simultaneously be used to understand the patient's values, goals, and meanings of illness, which should guide the personal and moral dimensions of the same process. In this instance, narrative theory was put into practice when the physician prompted Mr. B. and his daughter to describe their perception of Mrs. B.'s current condition, as well as how she has changed over recent years. The physician also shared his own perceptions. Reconciling the perceptions conveyed in these stories decisively shaped the process of medical decision making on Mrs. B.'s behalf.

This theory has some limitations. Consensus occurs in the context of choices. However, in the care of patients with severe dementia who live in nursing homes, local customs, beliefs, and systems of care can limit reasonable choices. For example, long-term-care regulations are often wrongly believed to require that all residents with severe swallowing difficulties receive artificial nutrition and hydration by initiating tube feeding. Surrogate-decision-maker laws are often misinterpreted to require a legally designated guardian for noncompetent patients who lack an advance directive.[4] Although a few state laws (in Missouri and New York) require a high degree of proof of a surrogate decision maker's knowledge of a patient's wishes to allow the surrogate to withhold or withdraw artificial hydration or nutrition from noncompetent patients, most states support the legal right of surrogate decision makers to refuse any and all unwanted medical treatments when this decision is based on a consensus of the patient's wishes and best interests.[4] In addition to legal inconsistencies and misperceptions, both health care systems and local community practices powerfully influence choices and decisions. For example, in the same community two otherwise high-quality nursing homes may have dramatically different rates of using feeding tubes for patients with severe dementia who develop swallowing difficulties. Research shows that large national variations in the rates of dying at home correlate with regional inpatient bed availability, not with patient or family preferences.[23]

An additional practical concern of a busy internist is that these dialogues take time. No empirical data compare the time requirements of this method with those of other decision-making strategies. However, investments in mutual understanding and trust building should ultimately improve decision making, promote higher-quality care, and prevent conflict as the patient's illness progresses.

"What happens if I feed her?" asks Mr. B. "Isn't she going to choke or get a worse pneumonia? Should we feed her by a tube or in her vein?"

Mr. B.'s questions describe a typical decision-making cascade. Typically, because oral feeding is thought to put the patient at risk for aspiration pneumonia, it is stopped. Mechanical feeding, either intravenously or enterally, is started so that the patient does not aspirate or starve.[10] At first blush, this seems like a logical thing to do. One can ensure adequate hydration and nutrition without taking the risk of aspiration of food into the lungs. Yet feeding tubes may not be as effective at preventing pneumonia as one might think, nor will it necessarily enhance the patient's quality or length of life.

Table 8–3 presents some of the benefits and burdens of feeding tubes for patients with dementia who develop significant difficulties swallowing. In addition to exploring the biomedical benefits and burdens of these technical interventions, the physician's duty is to explore other potential impacts of this intervention on the demented patient. Studies exploring the effects of feeding tubes on quality and length of life show mixed results. No randomized comparison of oral versus enteral feeding has been reported for this population of patients. Available studies suggest that enteral feeding does not significantly reduce, and may even increase, the risk of aspiration pneumonia.[17,24,25] In addition, enteral feeding may not prevent weight loss or the progression of pressure ulcers,[19,26,27] and is associated with substantial 1 year mortality rates.[28] Finally, a longitudinal cohort study[28] suggests that common nutritional compli-

TABLE 8–3. Potential Benefits and Burdens of Feeding Tubes in Patients with Severe Dementia Who Have Trouble Swallowing

BENEFITS	BURDENS
Biomedical	**Biomedical**
Improve hydration	Monitoring of metabolic status
Improve nutrition	Maintenance of tube
Careful monitoring of metabolic state	Primary focus on technical care
Potential to prolong life	Potential to prolong the dying process
Psychosocial	**Psychosocial**
Do "everything possible" to prolong life	Potential to prolong poor quality of life
Provide basic sense of care and feeding	Focus on technical aspects of care
Prevent perception of "starvation"	Lose smell and taste of real food
Make feeding quick and efficient	Lose human contact of feeding

cations of severe dementia can be managed by careful oral feeding. Given these data, the decision to use a feeding tube is best viewed as a personal choice based on deep values about the meaning of using a feeding tube or of continued oral feeding.

The physician explains that a feeding tube will allow the delivery of adequate nutrition and hydration for a woman of Mrs. B.'s age and weight, but it may not improve the quality or length of her life or prevent further aspiration. It may also deprive her of the tastes, smells, and touches of normal eating. He appeals to the family to recall how they just made the decision to care for Mrs. B.'s pneumonia. The key issue was the pleasure Mrs. B. received from her husband's daily visits and the food that he gave her.

The husband becomes agitated. "I just can't starve her, watch her starve, if that's what you're saying." He begins to weep.

"But Dad, she eats what she wants. No one's saying don't feed her. It's just don't force-feed her."

"But how will we know she's hungry?" he asks.

The physician offers a suggestion. "Her eating and your feeding her is one of the few meaningful activities that she has left. I think you both agree that we ought to at least allow her to try some food by mouth. Perhaps a speech therapist can give you some useful hints on feeding your wife. The issue of how best to feed your wife doesn't need to be made now. Let's take a few days and see how she does with both the pneumonia and the feeding. In between, don't hesitate to call me with any questions."

The dialogue has again reached a point of conflict. Table 4-3 in Chapter 4 lists some general ways to achieve common ground. In this case, the physician presents information about some of the burdens of enteral feeding and some of the benefits of continued oral feeding that had not been considered by the family. He then proposes a short-term trial of oral feeding, with the help of a speech therapist, while not precluding the possibility of enteral feeding in the future. In negotiating terms, he has proposed a compromise solution that avoids a power conflict and allows everyone's interests to be represented.

Two days later, Mrs. B.'s husband and daughter return. The husband explains, "I met with the therapist, and she showed me how to get her to eat a whole container of sherbet that she likes. We talked with our minister. I think we're going to keep it natural like that for now."

Mrs. B. gradually recovers from the pneumonia after several days of considerable physical distress (cough, respiratory distress, fever, and agitation). In addition to the oral antibiotics, her symptoms were palliated with opioids, humidified oxygen, nebulizers, antipyretic agents, and low-dose antipsychotic agents.

Several months pass. Mrs. B. is now unable to use a straw. Her intake of spoon-fed fluids and food is scant. Her husband worries that she will die of starvation. He and his daughter reapproach the physician for advice about how to proceed.

The physician, Mr. B., Mrs. B.'s daughter, and their minister review Mrs. B.'s life and recent events. After some discussion, the physician says, "Her Alzheimer's disease has progressed to the point where she's dying. I believe we ought to come up with a plan that minimizes her immediate suffering and maximizes her dignity and her quality of life."

A vigorous discussion follows. Eating was the one meaningful activity that remained in Mrs. B.'s life, but artificial feeding cannot serve the same function. Without that activity, the husband now believes that her quality of life is too poor to warrant the burdens of a feeding tube. Their minister agrees that a feeding tube would only prolong her suffering at this point. A plan is agreed upon to provide comfort measures only. She will be offered tastes and smells of her favorite foods and drinks; mouth and skin hygiene; lots of human contact, including repositioning and massage; but no enteral or intravenous nutrition or hydration.

After seven days, Mrs. B. dies.

Discussion

This case presents several common challenges to the practice of palliative care for patients with severe dementia. Mrs. B. could not speak for herself and, like most Americans, had not completed an advance directive. Even if she had, the preferences she expressed when competent may have been indeterminate guides for managing her actual problems. She could not tell us whether she was currently suffering or describe her present quality of life. The meaning of her signs and symptoms had to be interpreted. Furthermore, as a wife, mother, patient, and resident of a nursing home, she lived in a diverse community with many different views about what ought to be done for her. Finally, her problems included aspiration pneumonia and malnutrition as a consequence of swallowing difficulties that stemmed from her dementia. No randomized, controlled studies guide the provision of oral versus enteral feeding under these circumstances.[17-19,24-27] Despite this lack of evidence, those who care for and care about these patients must make decisions.

This case illustrates a palliative care strategy grounded in the theory that decisions for patients such as Mrs. B. are the result of dialogue and consensus building. The physician's initial investment of time may minimize the time and effort needed for future decisions. The physician's duty is to teach all participants that Mrs. B. has a chronic, irreversible, and ultimately fatal disease but also to learn from these participants about Mrs. B.'s values and quality of life. This frames decisions about hospitalization, antibiotics, and enteral nutritional support, medical choices that ultimately will shape the way she lives the last phase of her life.

As a result of this dialogue, a family may decide that continued efforts to prolong life are critical regardless of the severity of the patient's disease. Principles of negotiation that were outlined in Chapter 4 are often useful under these circumstances. In general, physicians should guide the discussion because of their familiarity with medical processes and prognoses, but surrogate decision makers must try to represent the patient's voice. Differences should be explored through dialogue that focuses on the patient's best interests and seeks common ground. Except when decisions seem to clearly violate the patient's best interests or prior wishes, the family has a final say in representing the patient in decision making. Families have to live with themselves and their role in these decisions long after the patient has died.

Conversely, some medical practitioners or long-term-care institutions see their primary job as prolonging life under all clinical circumstances because of religious principles or personal training. These practitioners or institutions should make their philosophy known from the outset, especially if they feel obligated to override the values and wishes of patients and families because they will be unable to pursue this consensus-based approach.

The meaning of suffering is personal and subjective. Evaluating the suffering of patients with dementia who cannot speak for themselves is inherently challenging. Even when suffering is recognized, its relief may be relegated in the pursuit of another goal, such as the preservation of life at all costs or hope for a miraculous cure. Through the process of repeatedly listening to the perspectives of each participant and involving the participants in a consensus-based interaction, decisions that respect the patient's dignity and quality of life can usually be achieved.

References

1. Doyle D, Hanks GW, MacDonald N. *Oxford Textbook of Palliative Medicine*, 2nd ed. New York: Oxford University Press, 1998.
2. Lo B, Dorbrand L. Guiding the hand that feeds. Caring for the demented elderly. *N Engl J Med* 1984; 311:402–404.
3. Meisel A. Barriers to forgoing nutrition and hydration in nursing homes. *Am J Law Med* 1995; 21:335–382.

4. Baile WF, DiMaggio JR, Schapira DV, Janofsky JS. The request for assistance in dying: The need for psychiatric consultation. *Cancer* 1993; 72:2786–2791.
5. Brock D. What is the moral authority of family members to act as surrogates for incompetent patients? *Milbank Q* 1996; 74:599–618.
6. Kuczewski MG. Reconceiving the family. The process of consent in medical decision-making. *Hastings Cent Rep* 1996; 26:30–37.
7. Brock D. Death and dying. In: Veatch RM, editor. *Medical Ethics*. Sudbury, Mass.: Jones and Bartlett, 1997.
8. Meisel A. *The Right to Die*, 2nd ed. New York: Wiley, 1995.
9. Buchanan A, Brock D. *Deciding for Others: The Ethics of Surrogate Decision Making*. Cambridge: Cambridge University Press, 1989.
10. Gillick MR. Rethinking the role of tube feeding in patients with advanced dementia. *N Engl J Med* 2000; 342:206–210.
11. Tulsky J, Fischer GS, Rose MR, Arnold RM. Opening the black box: how do physicians communicate about advance directives? *Ann Intern Med* 1998; 129:441–449.
12. The SUPPORT Principal Investigators. A controlled trial to improve care for seriously ill hospitalized patients. The study to understand prognoses and preferences for outcomes and risks of treatment (SUPPORT). *JAMA* 1995; 274: 1591–1598.
13. Virmani J, Schneiderman LJ, Kaplan RM. Relationship of advance directives to physician-patient communication. *Arch Intern Med* 1994; 154:909–913.
14. Rhymes J. Barriers to effective palliative care of terminal patients. Clin Ger Med 1996; 12:407–416.
15. Dresser R. Dworkin on dementia. Elegant theory, questionable policy. *Hastings Cent Rep* 1995; 25:32–38.
16. Schneiderman LJ, Jecker NS, Jonsen AR. Medical futility: its meaning and ethical implications. *Ann Intern Med* 1990; 112:949–954.
17. Prendergast TJ, Luce JM. Increasing incidence of withholding and withdrawal of life support from the critically ill. *Am J Respir Crit Care Med* 1997; 115:15–20.
18. Sulmasy DP, Terry PB, Weisman CS, Miller DJ, Stallings RY, Stallings RY. The accuracy of substituted judgments in patients with terminal diagnoses. *Ann Intern Med* 1998; 128:621–629.
19. Hurley AC, Volicer L, Rempusheski VF, Fry ST. Reaching consensus: the process of recommending treatment decisions for Alzheimer's patients. *Adv Nurs Sci* 1995; 18:33–43.
20. Quill TE, Brody H. Physician recommendations and patient autonomy: Finding a balance between physician power and patient choice. *Ann Intern Med* 1996; 125:763–769.
21. Hunter KM. *Doctors' Stories: The Narrative Structure of Medical Knowledge*. Princeton: Princeton University Press, 1991.
22. Bruner J. *Acts of Meaning*. Cambridge, MA: Harvard Univ Press, 1990.
23. Pritchard RS, Fisher ES, Teno J, Sharp SM, Reding DJ, Knaus WA, et al. Influence of patient preferences and local health system characteristics on the place of death. SUPPORT Investigators. Study to Understand Prognoses and Preferences for Risks and Outcomes of Treatment. *J Am Geriatr Soc* 1998; 46:1242–1250.
24. Ahronheim JC. Nutrition and hydration in the terminal patient. *Clin Geriatr Soc* 1996; 12:379–391.

25. Finucane TE, Bynum JP. Use of feeding tube to prevent aspiration pneumonia. *Lancet* 1996; 348:1421–1424.
26. Henderson CY, Trumbore LS, Mobarhan S, Benya R, Miles T. Prolonged tube feeding in long-term care: nutritional status and clinical outcome. *J Am Coll Nutr* 1992; 43:309–325.
27. Fincane TE. Malnutrition, feeding tubes and pressure sores: data are incomplete. *J Am Geriatr Soc* 1995; 43:447–451.
28. Volicer L, Selzer B, Rheaume Y, Karner J, Glennon M, Riley ME, et al. Eating difficulties in patients with probable dementia of the Alzheimer type. *J Geriatr Psychiatry Neurol* 1989; 2:188–195.

9

"Doctor, I Want to Die! Will You Help Me?"

It had been 18 months since Mr. K., a 67 year-old retired man, was diagnosed with inoperable lung cancer. An arduous course of chemotherapy helped him experience a relatively good year where he was able to remain independent, baby-sitting regularly for his two grandchildren, the main joys of his life.

Recent tests revealed new multiple bony metastases. An additional round of chemotherapy and radiation provided little relief. Over the ensuing three months, Mr. K.'s pain and fatigue became unrelenting. He was no longer able to tolerate, much less care for, his grandchildren. His wife of 45 years devoted herself to his care and support. Nevertheless, his days felt empty and his nights were dominated by despair about the future. Though he was treated with modern pain-control methods, his severe bone pain required daily choices between pain and sedation. Death was becoming less frightening than life itself.

A particularly severe episode of thigh pain led to a roentgenogram that showed circumferential destruction of his femur. Attempting to preserve his ability to walk, Mr. K. consented to the placement of a metal plate. Unfortunately, his bone was too brittle to support the plate. He would never walk again.

One evening in the hospital after his wife had just left, his physician sat down to talk to him. The pain was "about the same," and the new sleep medication "helped a little." He seemed quiet and distracted. When asked what was on his mind, Mr. K. looked directly at his doctor and said, "Doctor, I want to die. Will you help me?"

Such requests are dreaded by physicians. There is a desperate directness that makes sidestepping this question very difficult, if not impossible. By focusing mainly on the technology of care, physicians frequently avoid hearing about the inner turmoil faced by our terminally ill patients—what is happening to the person who has the disease. Yet sometimes requests for help in dying come from patients with strong wills, or out of desperation when there is nowhere else to turn. Though palliative care provides a humane alternative to traditional medical care of the dying,[1-7] it does not always provide guidance for how to approach those rare patients who continue to suffer terribly in spite of our best efforts. This chapter explores what dying patients might be experiencing when they make such requests and offers possible responses. Such discussions are by no means easy for clinicians, who may become exposed to forms and depths of suffering with which they are unfamiliar and to which they do not know how to respond. They may also fear being asked to violate their own moral standards or having to refuse someone in desperate need. Open exploration of requests for physician-assisted death can be fundamental to the humane care of a dying person; no matter how terrifying and unresolvable their suffering appears, at least they are no longer alone. Exploration also frequently opens up avenues of "help" that were not anticipated and that do not involve active assistance in dying.

"Doctor, I want to die" and "Will you help me?" are a statement and a query that must each be independently understood and explored. The physician's initial response, rather than a "yes" or "no" based on assumptions about the patient's intent and meaning, might be something like: "Of course I will try to help you, but first I need to understand your wish and your suffering, and then we can explore how I can help." Rather than shying away from the depths of suffering, follow-up questions might include "What is the worst part?" or "What is your biggest fear?"

The Wish to Die

Transient yearnings for death as an escape from suffering are common among patients with incurable, relentlessly progressive medical illnesses.[8-10] Such wishes are not necessarily signs of a psychiatric disorder, nor are they likely to be fully considered requests for a physician-assisted death. Let us explore some of their potential meanings through a series of case vignettes.

Tired of Acute Medical Treatment

A 55 year-old woman with very aggressive breast cancer found her tumor to be repeatedly recurring over six months. The latest instance signaled another failure of chemotherapy. As her doctor proposed a new round of experimental therapy, she said, "I wish I were dead." By exploring her statement, her physician learned that the patient felt strongly that she was not going to get better. She could not fathom the prospect of more chemotherapy with its side effects, and she wanted to spend what time she had left at home. He also learned that she did not want to die at that moment. A discussion about changing the goals of treatment from cure to comfort ensued, and a treatment plan was developed that exchanged chemotherapy for symptom-relieving treatments. The patient was relieved by this change in focus, and she was able to spend her last month at home with her family in a hospice program.

Palliative care can offer a caring and humane approach to the last phase of life by focusing energy on relieving the patients' suffering with the same intensity and creativity that traditional medical care usually devotes to treating underlying disease. When comprehensively applied, in a hospice program or any other setting, palliative care can help ensure a dignified, individualized death for most patients.

Unrecognized or Under-Treated Physical Symptoms

A stoic 85 year-old farmer with widely metastatic prostate cancer was cared for in his home with the help of a hospice program. Everyone marveled at his dry wit and engaging nature as he courageously faced death. He was taking very little medication and always said he was "fine." Everyone loved to visit with him, and his stories about life on the farm were legendary. As he became more withdrawn and caustic, people became concerned. When he said he wished he were dead, there was a panic. All the guns on the farm were hidden and plans for a psychiatric hospitalization were entertained. When his "wish for death" was fully explored, it turned out that he was living with excruciating pain, but not telling anyone because he feared becoming "addicted" to narcotics. After a long discussion about pain-relieving principles, the patient agreed to try a regular, around-the-clock dosage of long-acting opioid pain reliever with "as-needed" doses in between. In a short time, with his pain under better control, he again began to engage his family and visitors, and he no longer wanted to die. For the remainder of his life, physical symptoms that developed were addressed in a timely way, and he died a peaceful death surrounded by his family.

Though not all physical symptoms can be completely relieved by the creative application of palliative care, most can at least be made tolerable. New palliative techniques have been developed that can ameliorate most types of physical pain,[6,11–14] provided they are applied without unnecessary restraint. One must be sure that unrelieved symptoms are thoroughly explored, and that they are not a result of ignorance about available medical treatments, or of exaggerated fears about addiction or indirectly hastening death. Experts who can provide formal or informal consultation in pain control and in palliative care are accessible in most major cities, and extensive literature is available.

Emergent Psychosocial Problems

A 70 year-old retired woman with chronic leukemia that had become acute and had not responded to treatment was in a home hospice program. She was prepared to die, and all of her physicians felt that she would "not last more than a few weeks." She had lived alone in the past, but her daughter took a leave of absence from work to care for her mother for her last few days or weeks. Ironically (though not necessarily surprisingly), the woman stabilized at home. Two months later, outwardly comfortable and symptom-free under the supportive watch of her daughter, she began to focus on wanting to die. When asked to explain, she initially discussed her fatigue and her lack of a meaningful future. She then confided that she hated being a burden on her daughter. Her daughter had children who needed more of her attention and a job that was beginning to cause serious strain. The daughter had done her best to protect her mother from these problems, but she became aware of them anyway. A family meeting at which the problems were openly discussed resulted in a compromise whereby the mother was admitted to a nursing facility where comfort care was offered, and the daughter visited every other weekend. Though the mother would have liked to stay at home, she accepted this solution and lived for two more months before dying at the nursing facility with her daughter at her side.

Requests for help in dying can come about because of unrecognized or evolving psychosocial problems.[15] Sometimes these problems can be alleviated by having a family meeting, by arranging a temporary "respite" admission to a health care facility, or by consulting a social worker for advice about finances and available services. Other psychosocial problems may be more intractable— for example, in a family that was not functioning well prior to the patient's illness or when a dominating family member tries to influence care in a direction that appears contrary to the patient's wishes or best interest. Many patients have no family or financial resources. There are a growing number of volunteer-staffed, privately funded two-bed residential hospice units in most large communities that provide excellent palliative care for many who would otherwise fall through the cracks; however, the need for such units far exceeds their availability. Supplemental hospice services are also available in nursing homes, so excellent palliative care is available for many dying persons who cannot stay in their own home. Nevertheless, inadequate access to health care in general in the United States means that some dying patients who need the most help and support are forced to fend for themselves, and often die alone. The U.S. health care reimbursement system is primarily geared toward acute medical care, not terminal care, so a physician may be the only potential advocate and support that a dying patient has.

Spiritual Crisis

A 42 year-old woman who was living at home with advanced acquired immunodeficiency syndrome (AIDS) began saying that she wished she were dead. (The same patient is described in Chapter 6.) She was a fundamentalist Christian who at the time of her diagnosis wondered, "Why would God do this to me?" She eventually found meaning in the possibility that God was testing her strength, and that this was her "cross to bear." Although she continued to regularly participate in church activities for five years after her initial diagnosis, she never confided in her minister or church friends about her diagnosis. Her statements expressing her wish to be dead frightened her family, and they insisted she visit her doctor. When asked to elaborate on her wish, she raged against her church, her preacher, and God. She stated that she found her disease humiliating and did not want to be seen at the end stages of AIDS, when everyone would know. She felt more and more alone with these feelings, until she could no longer contain them. Once her feelings were acknowledged and understood, it was clear that they defied simple solution. She was legitimately angry, but not depressed. She had no real interest in taking her own life. She was eventually able to find a fundamentalist minister from a different church who had an open mind about AIDS and who helped her find spiritual consolation.

The importance of the physician's role as witness and support cannot be overemphasized. Sharing feelings of spiritual betrayal and uncertainty with an empathetic listener can be the first step toward healing. At least isolation is taken out of the doubt and despair. The physician must listen and try to fully understand the problem before making any attempt to help the patient achieve spiritual resolution. In many communities, medically experienced clergy are available who can explore spiritual issues with dying patients of many faiths so that isolation can be further lessened and the potential for reconnection with one's religious roots can be enhanced.

Clinical Depression

A 60 year-old man with a recently diagnosed recurrence of non-Hodgkin's lymphoma became preoccupied with wanting to die. Though he had a long remission after his first course of chemotherapy, he had recently gone through a divorce and felt he could not face more treatment. It became evident that he was preoccupied with thoughts of his father, who had gone through an agonizing death filled with severe pain and agitation. He had a strong premonition that the same thing would happen to him, and he was not sleeping because of this worry. He appeared withdrawn, and he was not able to fully understand that odds suggested treatment directed at his lymphoma would be successful. He also had trouble comprehending the likelihood that palliative care could prevent a death like his father's, despite his doctor's promise to work with him to find acceptable solutions. Although he was thinking seriously of suicide, he did not have a plan for ending his life, and therefore he was treated intensively as an outpatient by his internist and a psychotherapist. He accepted the idea that he was depressed, but he also wanted assurances that all possibilities for easing his death could be explored after a legitimate trial of treatment for depression. He responded well to a combination of psychotherapy and medication, and eventually he underwent acute treatment directed at his lymphoma that unfortunately did not work. He then requested hospice care and seemed comfortable and engaged in his last months. As death approached, his symptoms remained relatively well controlled, and he was not overtly depressed. He died alone while his family was out of the house. Since his recently filled prescription bottles were all empty, it may have been a drug overdose (presumably to avoid an end like his father's).

Whenever a severely ill person begins to talk about wanting to die, and begins to seriously consider taking his or her own life, the question of clinical depression appropriately arises.[8,16–18] This can be a complex and delicate determination, because most patients who are near death with unrelenting suffering are very sad, if not clinically depressed. Many of the symptoms of terminal illness are also associated with depression (fatigue, weight loss, sleep disturbance, preoccupation with death), so usual symptom-based depression scales tend to over-report the incidence of depression in the terminally ill. Studies using modified depression scales that avoid this potential for over-reporting still show a higher incidence of depression in the terminally ill than that in nonterminal controls (13% measured by modified scales versus 26.1% measured by normal criteria),[17,19] yet there is a growing clinical literature suggesting that some of these suicides are rational.[2,20–24]

Two fundamental questions must be answered before suicide can be considered rational in such settings: (1) Is the patient able to fully understand his or her disease, prognosis, and treatment alternatives (i.e., is the decision rational)? and (2) Is the patient's depression reversible, given the limitations imposed by his or her illness, to an extent that would substantially alter the patient's situation? It is vital not to over-normalize (e.g., "anyone would be depressed under such circumstances") or to reflexively define a request for death as a sign of psychopathology. Each patient's dilemma must be fully explored individually. Consultation with an experienced psychiatrist can be helpful when there is doubt about a diagnosis or its implications. For a potentially reversible depression, most experts recommend at least a trial of amphetamines[25-27] or other antidepressant medications if the patient has the time and strength for such treatment.

Unrelenting, Intolerable Suffering

Mr. K., the retired man with widely metastatic lung cancer described in the introduction of this chapter, felt that his life had become a living hell with no acceptable options. His doctors agreed that all effective medical options to treat his cancer had been exhausted. Physical activity and pride in his body had always been a central part of who he was. Now, with a pathologic fracture in his femur that could not be repaired, he would not even be able to walk independently. He also had to make daily trade-offs between pain, sedation, and other side effects. At the insistence of his doctor, he met with a psychiatrist several times who found his judgment to be fully rational. Death did not appear imminent, and his condition could only get worse. Even in a hospice program, with experts doing their best to help address his medical, social, personal, and spiritual concerns, he felt trapped, yearning for death. He saw his life savings from 45 years of work rapidly depleting. His family offered to supplement his finances and to provide additional personal support. They wanted him to live, but having witnessed his last months of progressive disability, loss, and pain, with no relief in sight other than death, they eventually decided to respect his wishes and gradually started to advocate on his behalf: "We appreciate your efforts to keep him comfortable, but for him this is not comfortable and it is not living. Will you help him?"

Physicians who have made a commitment to shepherd their patients through the dying process find themselves in a predicament. They can acknowledge that standard palliative care is sometimes far less than ideal but it is the best that they can offer. Alternatively, they can search with the patient and family for assistance in dying that is agreeable to all parties. Some of these methods are explored in detail in Chapter 12. Compassionate physicians differ widely in their approach to this dilemma,[21,22,24,28-31] though most support openly discussing death with a patient who raises the issue and an extensive search for alternative approaches.

Clinical criteria have been proposed to guide physicians who find assisted suicide a morally acceptable last-resort option:[24,32,33]

1. The patient must, of his or her own free will and at his or her own initiative, clearly and repeatedly request to die rather than continue suffering.
2. The patient's judgment must not be distorted.
3. The patient must have a condition that is incurable and associated with severe, unrelenting, intolerable suffering.
4. The physician must ensure that the patient's suffering and the request are not the result of inadequate palliative care.
5. Any of the interventions described in Chapter 12 that can end in a patient's death should be carried out only in the context of a meaningful doctor–patient relationship.
6. Consultation with another physician who is experienced in end-of-life care is required.
7. Clear documentation to support each condition above should be required (physician-assisted suicide, because of its ambiguous legal status outside of Oregon, is the exception; nevertheless, all conditions should be carefully evaluated and met).

It is not the purpose of this chapter to review the public policy implications of society's formally accepting these criteria or of maintaining current prohibitions. Instead, it is to encourage and guide clinicians on both sides of the issue to openly explore the possible meanings of a patient's request for help in dying and to search as widely as possible for acceptable responses that are tailored to the needs of the individual patient.

The Request for Help in Dying

All dying patients need more than prescriptions for opioids and referrals to hospice programs from their physicians, and those who express a wish to die certainly need more than a prescription for barbiturates. Instead, such patients need a personal guide and counselor throughout the dying process —someone who will unflinchingly help them face both the medical and the personal aspects of dying, whether they go smoothly or take the physician into unfamiliar, untested ground.[34] Dying patients do not have the luxury of choosing not to undertake the journey, or of separating their person from their disease. Physicians' commitment not to abandon their patients is of paramount importance.[35]

Fears about dying badly usually first emerge when someone is diagnosed with a life-threatening illness, or when a patient's illness has gone through a major exacerbation and the prognosis is uncertain. Under these circumstances, patients and their family members begin to consider what their future might look like. As part of that inquiry, they may imagine the "worst-case scenario." Patients may not have to look very far if they have witnessed a bad death in their own family or with close friends. In addition to exploring a patient's hopes for the future, a clinician should also inquire about the patient's fears. After carefully listening to the patient's response, the clinician should further explore these fears, if possible using the patient's own language, so that the patient feels heard and understood.

DOCTOR: *As you look to the future, what are your biggest fears?*

PATIENT: *I am not afraid of pain, but I am afraid of dying out of my mind.*

DOCTOR: *Tell me more about what you mean by "dying out of my mind."*

PATIENT: *I saw my father die that way, and it was awful. He was such a refined man, and to see him die screaming, hallucinating, and completely out of control was excruciating!*

DOCTOR: *That sounds like it must have been terrible, both for him and the rest of the family.*

PATIENT: *We all felt horrible, like we really let him down.*

Only after fully exploring the patient's experience, including its associated emotions, can the clinician begin to be genuinely reassuring. Table 9–1 shows some simple techniques for responding to a patient's emotions.[36]

TABLE 9–1. Levels of Responding to Emotion

RESPONSE	ILLUSTRATIVE QUESTION
• Acknowledge	• *"I can see you find this distressing."*
	• *"You seem very sad today."*
• Legitimize	• *"Anyone in your shoes would be upset."*
	• *"It seems only natural to be angry about the way things turned out."*
• Explore	• *"What is the most distressing part?"*
	• *"Tell me more about what is making you angry (sad, nervous, upset)."*
• Empathize	• *"That sounds terrifying."*
	• *"I imagine I would feel overwhelmed too."*

If a patient's main fear is of pain, particularly if prior physicians have been reluctant to prescribe adequate amounts of opioid analgesics, clinicians should respond in a way that will relieve the patient's concerns. (*"We now can adequately relieve almost all kinds of pain. I have no reservations about prescribing adequate amounts of opioids. If you have a lot of pain in the future, we will work together until you tell me your pain is sufficiently relieved."*) A patient who has witnessed other symptoms, such as severe shortness of breath or an agitated delirium, may be more difficult to reassure. Under these circumstances, the patient may need some ideas about how the physician approaches both the specific problem in question and a more open-ended commitment.

DOCTOR: *Most of the time, the difficulties associated with dying can be made quite tolerable by using well-described techniques developed in hospice and palliative care, but managing severe agitation and confusion like what happened with your father can be difficult. When all else fails in such circumstances, we now heavily sedate such patients so they can escape from this kind of agony. I can promise that I and the rest of our team will do our best to work with you to face whatever has to be faced.*

PATIENT: *I wish that kind of an escape could have been available to my father.*

DOCTOR: *I wish it could have been too. We have come a long way in terms of our abilities to address severe forms of suffering.*

A commitment to see the dying process through is fundamental,[35] and needs to be articulated even if the patient does not bring it up. Whether patients choose to engage in an aggressive fight for life using intensive medical technology, or transition to an approach that emphasizes palliation, or anything in between, they need a committed medical partner.

DOCTOR: *I want to let you know that we are in this together. No matter what happens, I will work with you to find the best approach possible.*

Some patients ask pointed and difficult questions about the nature and extent of their physician's future commitment, including the possibility of actively helping the patient to die. Rather than provide a quick answer based on personal values and experience, the physician may be well-advised to probe further by asking what kind of "help" the patient is asking about. (*"When you say 'help me to die,' I am not exactly sure what kind of 'help' you are talking about."*) Many patients simply ask for assurance that they will receive all the pain medications they may need, whereas others look for an open-ended commitment from the physician to face the unknown with them. The clinician should base his or her response with regard to methods on exactly what is being requested by the patient.

If the patient asks about medication that could be used for a physician-assisted suicide, the clinician should discuss this possibility in the proper context, as long as he or she is willing to provide this option.

DOCTOR: *I know how important the possibility of an escape is to you as you contemplate your future. Because palliative care is so effective, my experience is that physician-assisted suicide is rarely needed. We will use all means possible to alleviate your pain and suffering, but if those measures prove ineffective or unacceptable, I will explore this possibility with you as a very last resort.*

A clinician who cannot provide this option because of personal, moral, or legal constraints should say so unhesitatingly, but also reassure the patient that this need not affect the nature and depth of their commitment. This response might also include an exploration of the last-resort options the clinician can provide under the circumstances feared by the patient:

DOCTOR: *I know that the possibility of an escape is important to you, but I personally cannot provide medication that could be used in an overdose. I believe that palliative care is very effective, and that we can address most kinds of suffering. However, if your situation becomes intolerable to you, I will work with you to try to find an acceptable answer. If all else fails, I would even be willing to provide heavy sedation, so that you would be unaware of your suffering.*

Most palliative care clinicians find that such open discussion, a commitment to see the process through, and a willingness to seek creative solutions to difficult forms of terminal suffering are more fundamental to a patient's well-being than a simple willingness to prescribe or not prescribe barbiturates.

Armed with such an open-ended commitment from their physician, including a promise to address their worst fears if they materialize, most patients feel more secure and free to bring peaceful resolution to their lives. They are in a position very different from that of patients and families who do not have a medical partner they can count on under any circumstances. Knowledge that there *could be* an escape is important to many, but in actuality, few will ever need it.

Requests for assistance in dying rarely evolve into fully considered requests for physician-assisted suicide. As illustrated in the case vignettes, a thorough exploration of the patient's experience and the immediate reason for the request often yield avenues of "help" that are acceptable to patients, families, physicians, and ethicists.

The clinical summaries in this chapter have been over-simplified to illustrate particular issues. More commonly, multiple issues and patient motives exist simultaneously, perhaps yielding several opportunities for intervention. The first step is to understand why the patient's suffering has become so unbearable right now (*"First I need to learn more about why your suffering has become so unacceptable right now." "What is the worst part?" "Why is it worse now than last week or last month?"*).

TABLE 9–2. Sources of Reversible Suffering That May Lead to Requests for a Physician-Assisted Death

DIMENSION OF SUFFERING	QUESTION TO INITIATE EXPLORATION
• Tired of acute medical treatment	• *"I can see that the treatment is not working very well, and that it has been very hard on you. Perhaps it is time to focus our energy more exclusively on your quality of life and comfort. Have you heard about hospice programs?"*
• Unrecognized or under-treated physical symptoms	• *"Sometimes people are having pain or other uncomfortable symptoms that they don't talk about. These symptoms may be very responsive to treatment. Are you having any such problems that we have not addressed?"*
• Emergent psychosocial problems	• *"Sometimes even the most caring families get tired out by the challenges of caregiving, especially with the demands of modern life. Are you and your family having any difficulties? Are there issues with any particular family members that are worrying you?* *How about financial problems?"*
• Spiritual crisis	• *"Sometimes people who are as sick as you are have a crisis of faith—like wondering how God could do this to you. Have you had any similar concerns? Are there any spiritual or religious matters that have been left unaddressed?"*
• Clinical depression (or other mental disorder)	• *"Are you depressed?"(46) "Do you have feelings of hopelessness or despair? Are there any things that you can still enjoy? How do you see the future?"*

Potential dimensions of suffering that should be explored and evaluated are presented in Table 9–2, along with sample questions to begin an inquiry.[37,38] Usually these interviews include close family members who may have insight into the patient's clinical situation and ideas about alternative approaches. Of course, the patient is the ultimate arbiter of who gets included as "family" in these conversations.

What Do Dying Persons Want Most From Their Physicians?

Most patients do not want to die, but if they must, they would like to do it while maintaining their physical and personal integrity.[39] When faced with a patient expressing a wish for death and a request for help, physicians (and others) should consider the following:

1. *Listen and Learn from the Patient before Responding*

   Learning as much as possible about the patient's unique suffering and about exactly what is being requested is a vital first step. Physicians tend to be action oriented, yet these problems only infrequently yield simple solutions. This is not to say they are insoluble, but the patient is the initial guide to defining the problem and the range of acceptable interventions.

2. *Be Compassionate, Caring, and Creative*

   Palliative care is a far cry from "not doing anything." It is completely analogous to intensive medical care, but the care is directed toward a person and his or her suffering, not a disease. Dying patients need our commitment to creatively problem-solve, and our support no matter where their illness may go. Rules and methods are not simple when applied to real persons, but the satisfaction derived from helping someone find his or her own path to a dignified death can be immeasurable.

3. *Promise to Be There Until the End*

   Many people have personally witnessed or in some way encountered "bad deaths," though this might mean different things to different people. Patients need our assurance that if things get undignified or intolerable we will not abandon them and we will continue to work with them to find acceptable solutions. Usually those solutions do not involve directly helping a patient to die, but they often involve aggressive use of symptom-relieving measures that might indirectly hasten death.[3,40] We should be able to reassure all of our patients that they will not die racked by physical pain, for it is now accepted practice to give increasing amounts of analgesic medicine until the pain is relieved, even if it inadvertently shortens a life. Many patients find this promise reassuring, for it both alleviates their fear of pain and provides proof of the physician's willingness to find creative, aggressive solutions.

4. *If Asked, Be Honest About Your Openness to the Possibility (or Impossibility) of Physician-Assisted Suicide*

   Many patients who want to explore their physicians' willingness to provide a potentially lethal prescription fear being out of control, physically dependent, or mentally incapacitated, rather than physical pain alone.[41–44] For many, the possibility of a controlled death if their pain or situation becomes intolerable is often more important than the reality. Those who secretly hold lethal prescriptions or who have a physician who will entertain the possibility of such treatment feel a sense of control knowing that, if things become intolerable, they have a potential escape. Other patients are assured simply by knowing that we can acknowledge the problem, talk about death, and actively search for acceptable approaches, even if we cannot directly help them to die. Chapter 12 explores important alternatives to physician-assisted suicide for all patients and physicians.

5. *Approach Intolerable End-of-Life Suffering with an Open Heart and an Open Mind*

   Though acceptable solutions can almost always be found through the skillful application of state-of-the-art palliative care principles, this is not a time for denial of the problem or for superficial solutions. If there are no good alternatives, what should the patient do? There is often a moment of truth for health care providers and families faced with a patient who has no acceptable options. Physicians must not turn their backs, but instead must continue to problem-solve, to be present, and to help their patients find dignity in death.

6. *Do Not Forget Your Own Support*

   Working with dying patients can be both enriching and emotionally draining. It forces clinicians to face their own mortality, abilities, and limitations. It is vital to have a place to openly share grief and uncertainties, as well as to take joy in small victories.[45] For us to deepen our understanding of the human condition and to help humanize the dying process for our patients and ourselves, we must learn to give voice to and share our experience of working closely with dying patients.

The patients with whom we engage at this level often become indelibly imprinted on our identities as medical professionals. Much like the death of a family member, the process that they go through and our willingness and ability to be there and to be helpful are often replayed and rethought. The intensity of these relationships and our ability to make a difference are often without parallel. This road is eventually traveled by all of us. However, the map is poorly described and the journey unpredictable, frequently making for an adventure with extraordinary richness but unclear boundaries.

- *Note*: Many of the ideas and cases presented in this chapter were initially presented in an article I wrote titled "Doctor, I want to die. Will you help me?" published in the *Journal of the American Medical Association* 1993; 270:870–873.

References

1. Wanzer SH, Adelstein SJ, Cranford RE, Federman DD, Hook ED, Moertel CG, et al. The physician's responsibility toward hopelessly ill patients. *N Engl J Med* 1984; 310:955–959.
2. Wanzer SH, Federman DD, Adelstein SJ, Cassel CK, Cassem EH, Cranford RE, et al. The physician's responsibility toward hopelessly ill patients: A second look. *N Engl J Med* 1989; 320:844–849.
3. American Medical Association's Council on Ethical and Judicial Affairs. Decisions near the end of life. *JAMA* 1992; 276:2229–2233.

4. Rhymes J. Hospice care in America. *JAMA* 1990; 264:369–372.
5. Hastings Center. (1987). *Guidelines on the Termination of Life-Sustaining Treatment and the Care of the Dying*. New York: The Hastings Center.
6. Doyle D, Hanks GW, MacDonald N. *Oxford Textbook of Palliative Medicine*, 2nd ed. New York: Oxford University Press, 1998.
7. Quill TE. *Death and Dignity: Making Choices and Taking Charge*. New York: W.W. Norton and Co., 1993.
8. Chochinov HM, Wilson KG, Enns M, Mowchun N, Lander S, Levitt M, et al. Desire for death in the terminally ill. *Am J Psychiatry* 1995; 152:1185–1191.
9. Breitbart W, Rosenfeld BD, Passik SD. Interest in physician-assisted suicide among ambulatory HIV-infected patients. *Am J Psychiatry* 1996; 153:238–242.
10. Emanuel EJ, Fairclough DL, Daniels ER, Clarridge BR. Euthanasia and physician-assisted suicide: attitudes and experiences of oncology patients, oncologists, and the public. *Lancet* 1996; 347:1805–1810.
11. Foley KM. The treatment of cancer pain. *N Engl J Med* 1989; 313:84–95.
12. Kane RL, Bernstein L, Wales J, Rothenberg R. Hospice effectiveness in controlling pain. *JAMA* 1985; 253:2683–2686.
13. Twycross RG, Lack SA. *Symptom Control in Far Advanced Cancer*. London: Pitman Books, 1983.
14. Kerr IG, Sone M, DeAngelis C, Iscoe N, MacKenzie R, Schueller T. Continuous narcotic infusion with patient-contolled analgesia for chronic cancer pain in out-patients. *Ann Intern Med* 1988; 108:554–557.
15. Garfield CA. *Psychosocial Care of the Dying Patient*. New York: McGraw-Hill Book Company, 1978.
16. Conwell Y, Caine ED. Rational suicide and the right to die—reality and myth. *N Engl J Med* 1991; 325:1100–1103.
17. Chochinov HM, Wilson KG, Enns M, Lander S. Prevalence of depresson in the terminally ill: Effects of diagnostic criteria and symptom threshold judgments. *Am J Psychiatry* 1994; 151:537–540.
18. Block SD. Assessing and managing depression in the terminally ill patient. ACP-ASIM End-of-Life Care Consensus Panel. *Ann Intern Med* 2000; 132:209–218.
19. Kathol RG, Noyes R Jr, Williams J, Mutgi A, Carroll B, Perry P. Diagnosing depression in patients with medical illness. *Psychosomatics* 1990; 31:434–440.
20. Cassel CK, Meier DE. Morals and moralism in the debate over euthanasia and assisted suicide. *N Engl J Med* 1990; 323:750–752.
21. Quill TE. Death and dignity: A case of individualized decision making. *N Engl J Med* 1991; 324:691–694.
22. Jecker NS. Giving death a hand: when the dying and the doctor stand in a special relationship. *J Am Geriatr Sac* 1991; 39:831–835.
23. Angell M. Euthanasia. *N Engl J Med* 1988; 319:1348–1350.
24. Brody H. Assisted death—a compassionate response to a medical failure. *N Engl J Med* 1992; 327:1384–1385.
25. Woods SW, Tesar GE, Murray GB, Cassem NH. Psychostimulant treatment of depressive disorders secondary to medical illness. *J Clin Psychiatry* 1986; 1986:12–15.
26. Masand P, Pickett P, Murray GB. Psychostimulants for secondary depression in medical illness. *Psychosomatics* 1991; 32:203–208.
27. Burns MM, Eisendrath SJ. Dextroamphetamine treatment for depression in terminally ill patients. *Psychosomatics* 1994; 35:80–83.
28. Angell M. The quality of mercy. *N Engl J Med* 1982; 306:98–99.

29. Singer PA, Siegler M. Euthanasia—a critique. *N Engl J Med* 1975; 292:78–80.
30. Gaylin W, Kass LR, Pellegrino ED, Siegler M. "Doctors must not kill." *JAMA* 1988; 259:2139–2140.
31. Gomez C. *Regulating Death: Euthanasia and the Case of the Netherlands*. New York, NY: Free Press, 1991.
32. Quill TE, Cassel CK, Meier DE. Care of the hopelessly ill. Proposed criteria for physician-assisted suicide. *N Engl J Med* 1992; 327:1380–1384.
33. Baron CH, Bergstresser C, Brock DW, Cole GF, Dorfman NS, Johnson JA, et al. Statute: A model state act to authorize and regulate physician-assisted suicide. *Harvard Journal on Legislation* 1996; 33:1–34.
34. Quill TE. *A Midwife Through the Dying Process. Stories of Healing and Hard Choices at the End of Life*. Baltimore: Johns Hopkins University Press, 1996.
35. Quill TE, Cassel CK. Nonabandonment: A central obligation for physicians. *Ann Intern Med* 1995; 122:368–374.
36. Novack DH. Therapeutic aspects of the clinical encounter. *J Gen Intern Med* 1987; 2:346–355.
37. Block SD, Billings JA. Patient requests to hasten death: Evaluation and management in terminal care. *Arch Intern Med* 1994; 154:2039–2047.
38. Emanuel LL. Facing requests for physician-assisted suicide. *JAMA* 1998; 280: 643–647.
39. Cassell EJ. *The Nature of Suffering and the Goals of Medicine*. New York: Oxford University Press, 1991.
40. Quill TE, Lo B, Brock DW. Palliative options of last resort: A comparison of voluntarily stopping eating and drinking, terminal sedation, physician-assisted suicide, and voluntary active euthanasia. *JAMA* 1997; 278:1099–2104.
41. Back AL, Wallace JI, Starks HE, Pearlman RA. Physician-assisted suicide and euthanasia in Washington State: Patient requests and physician responses. *JAMA* 1996; 275:919–925.
42. Chin AE, Hedberg K, Higginson GK, Fleming DW. Legalized physician-assisted suicide in Oregon—the first year's experience. *N Engl J Med* 1999; 340(7):577–583.
43. van der Maas PJ, van Delden JJM, Pijnenborg L. The Remmelink Study. *Health Policy* 1992; 22.
44. van der Maas PJ, van der Wal G, Haverkate I, de Graaff CL, Kester JG, Onwuteaka-Philipsen BD, et al. Euthanasia, physician-assisted suicide, and other medical practices involving the end of life in the Netherlands, 1990–1995. *N Engl J Med* 1996; 335:1699–1705.
45. Quill TE, Williamson P. Healthy approaches to physician stress. *Arch Intern Med* 1990; 150:1857–1861.
46. Chochinov HM, Wilson KG, Enns M, Lander S. "Are you depressed?" Screening for depression in the terminally ill. *Am J Psychiatry* 1997; 154:674–676.

10

Hospice and Palliative Care: Clinical, Ethical, and Policy Challenges

Palliative care is defined as the biological, psychological, social, and spiritual care of patients whose diseases are not responsive to curative treatment.[1] The goal of palliative care is to provide the best possible quality of life for both the patient and the family. Palliative care should be provided to all seriously ill and dying patients, whether or not they are still actively involved in treating their underlying diseases. In the United States, hospice refers to a Medicare-sponsored program to provide palliative care for terminally ill patients and their families. Hospice, the "cadillac" of comprehensive home care programs, provides a high standard of excellence in the care of the dying. Hospice in Great Britain usually represents a residential place where terminally ill patients are provided comprehensive palliative care for the last months of their lives.

Medicare-financed hospice programs operate under restrictions that make them unavailable to many dying patients.[2] To qualify, patients must have a prognosis of six months or less with a high level of certainty, and must be willing to forgo aggressive treatment of their underlying diseases. Hospice programs provide the support of a multidisciplinary team, including nurses, social workers, clergy, physical therapists, nutritionists, volunteers, and a physician consultant. Every effort is made to assist family members in the care of the patient at home. Admission to an acute hospital or palliative care inpatient unit for management of severe symptoms is provided, as well as respite care under certain circumstances. Medicare imposes some restrictions on the average percentage of inpatient days each year for all patients enrolled in a hospice program, but these limits are rarely reached. In addition to supporting patients and families at home, hospice programs can now supplement care in nursing homes. There are also a growing number of small hospice houses where volunteers operate as family for patients who do not have a suitable home environment. Hospice programs are required to have 24-hour availability of emergency support services through an on-call system, usually staffed by highly trained palliative care nurses. Hospice also provides bereavement care for family members after a patient's death.

Using the knowledge and skills of their multidisciplinary teams, hospices are effective at controlling most pain and symptoms, and at giving patients and their families the opportunity to prepare for death in a manner consistent with their personal goals and values.[3] Most patients and family members evaluate their experience on hospice programs positively, and recommend the experience to others in the same situation. Dying may not be something to look forward to, but if we have to die, such programs allow us to make the most of a potentially difficult situation.

To illustrate how hospice works, two patients will be presented. Both needed and received palliative care, but they had unequal access to formal hospice programs. Both benefited from palliative care interventions, but each found some limitations to the degree of palliation and support they received during periods of their illnesses. Both patients also had difficult-to-manage symptoms at times, and both wanted a mix of disease-related intervention and palliative care that did not fit with the Medicare hospice benefit. Furthermore, they varied considerably in their desire and willingness to address the "developmental issues" of dying. I present these cases both to illustrate the potential effectiveness of palliative care and to show that the clinical, ethical, and policy dilemmas are complex and at times vexing even under the guidance of a skilled team of caregivers.

Mr. B.

Mr. B. was a 70 year-old Italian-American who already had widely metastatic prostate cancer when I first met him. I had cared for several members of his family and knew about his illness based on preexisting conversations, but I had never personally met or cared for Mr. B. until his disease was extremely advanced. His cancer had been effectively suppressed by experimental therapy for the last year, but it was no longer controlling the pain stemming from increasing bony metastases and the fever emanating from liver metastases. Although he was reluctant about accepting morphine (which he saw as a sign of impending death), he wanted his symptoms to be better controlled so he could spend more quality time with his children and grandchildren. His biggest fear about the future was uncontrolled pain, and I was able to reassure him that I would have no restraints about offering him as much pain medicine as he might require if the need arose in the future.

Mr. B. knew that his disease was very advanced, but he was not prepared to accept death as inevitable, and he wanted to see if any further experimental therapies could be found that might work without making him more symptomatic in the process. Since the odds of his responding to experimental therapy were very low, and the odds of his dying in the next six months were very high, I raised the possibility of his entering a home hospice program. We could then devote all of our energy to keeping him comfortable and enhancing the meaning of his remaining life. He appreciated the offer, and said he would keep it "in his back pocket" should his situation and goals change in the future. For now, however, he was not prepared to accept a six-month prognosis, nor was he willing to give up on aggressive disease-related therapy that had any chance of prolonging his life. At my suggestion, he agreed to forgo cardiopulmonary resuscitation (CPR) because it was very invasive and extremely unlikely to be successful given his burden of disease. A home do-not-resuscitate (DNR) order was written to guide ambulance crews should he suffer a cardiac arrest at home. Any and all other potentially effective treatments would be jointly considered by Mr. B., his children, and me as his physician.

Although this decision to pursue aggressive treatment precluded his being admitted to a formal hospice program (for which he would otherwise have qualified), it did not mean that we would not work intensively to relieve his pain and fever and enhance his quality of life. I assured Mr. B that taking regular doses of opioid pain medication in no way meant giving in to his disease or death, and that better pain management would allow him to have more energy for his family, which was his primary goal. We were also able to bring his fever down with nonsteroidal anti-inflammatory medications. We agreed that if his disease responded to experimental therapy, any of the palliative treatments that were no longer needed would be discontinued.

In consultation with his oncologist, we found a chemotherapy regimen that sounded promising and was not likely to be toxic. Of course, "promising" was at most temporary suppression of his disease and not a cure, but this was enough for Mr. B. to take a chance. At the same time, his pain and fever abated with long-acting morphine tablets taken regularly along with the nonsteroidal anti-inflammatories, so he was able to experience life with his family more fully. He began to visit his family members at their homes instead of having them come to his apartment. For Mr. B., this was a giant step forward in terms of independence and well-being. Mr. B. was cautiously optimistic, but he knew that his condition was fragile, and that any day he might be dealing with matters of life and death. For now, however, he chose to ignore explicit exploration of his vulnerable situation as much as possible, and to live life fully in the present.

Because Mr. B. was knowledgeable about his condition, he did not waste time on trivial matters. He was not in denial; he simply chose to focus all of his available psychological and spiritual energy on his family. Yet the time he spent with his children and grandchildren was much more likely to include conversation about their schoolwork or the most recent Yankee game than any deep existential exchange. This was Mr. B.'s way. Most of his medical visits were attended by one or two of his children. If it appeared that his disease was progressing, he would ask that they leave the room, and he would ask me direct questions about his prognosis. He wanted honest answers about how much time I thought he had, and whether it made any sense to continue with the chemotherapy. He did not ask a lot of questions, but those he did ask were to the point, reflecting a deep understanding of his disease and future. With Mr. B.'s permission, I would then report these conversations to his children, but they did not discuss these issues explicitly with one another. Offers to facilitate more direct conversation were politely rejected—the children felt such exchanges would be too painful for all concerned. I became a go-between to keep everyone informed, which seemed to work for this particular family.

Several months later, Mr. B. suddenly stopped being able to eat and drink, and simultaneously he developed severe pain in his upper abdomen. He was admitted to our palliative care inpatient unit for evaluation and acute symptom management. The mucous membranes in Mr. B.'s mouth were raw and bleeding, and we decided to take a direct look at his esophagus and stomach with a fiber-optic endoscope in hopes of finding something easily reversible. Fortunately, we identified an ulcer and a severe yeast infection that accounted for his symptoms, which improved dramatically with a combination of stomach acid suppression and antifungal treatment. We also used the opportunity that this hospitalization provided to see if the chemotherapy was suppressing his cancer sufficiently to warrant the risk of further aggravating his stomach condition.

The answer was not unexpected: His cancer was progressing on all fronts, showing up in blood serological markers as well as tests of his liver and bones. Experimental chemotherapy now made no sense, and there were no other aggressive measures with any realistic chance of affecting his disease. After privately apprising Mr. B. of his clinical situation, we had a family meeting where we discussed transitioning into a formal hospice program. The level of support that could be provided at home would be increased, and his medication would all be paid for by the program. Based on similar cases, his prognosis was six months or less, though there was always the possibility that he would be an exception. ("You have already been the exception in so many ways!") All efforts would be made to keep him comfortable and at home; his large family would rotate visiting on a fixed schedule. If he developed major problems in the future, he could always return to the palliative care unit at the hospital for more intensive symptom management.

Mr. B.'s symptoms of pain and fever were initially well-controlled. His family (children, grandchildren, siblings, and others) all visited regularly. Ball games were watched together, family photos were reminisced about, and cards were played. There was very little explicit acknowledgment of his dying, other than a few side conversations during which I would inform Mr. B. and then his family about any change in his disease progression or prognosis. The hospice nurse visited weekly, but he had no needs for home health aides with respect to personal care. He was visited by his own priest, who found no major spiritual or religious matters that needed settling. At first he came to the office to see me, and then, as he became weaker, I went to see him at his home.

Mr. B. became weaker and more dependent on others. He occasionally needed to be toileted by his sons and daughter. As much as he hated accepting help from his family, personal care by strangers was even less acceptable. He found this level of weakness and dependence humiliating, and no amount of reassurance by his children made it acceptable to him. We tried to "reframe" the experience as a chance for his children to give care back to a man who had given them so much, but he never made peace with his dependence on others for personal care. His pain and fever were well controlled, but to him his progressive weakness and debility were his most disturbing symptoms.

As death approached, his pain suddenly got worse. I assessed him at home and found the pain to be diffuse and severe, stemming mainly from his extensive bone metastases. We talked about an unusual radioactive treatment that might be effective at relieving his pain, but Mr. B. now wanted no further technologic interventions. He was prepared for death, and he wanted to be out of pain even if he had to be sedated. I ordered progressive increases in both his around-the-clock and "as needed" pain medications. He remained in agony for the next 12 hours, and requested a return to the palliative care inpatient unit. We readmitted him, and were able to adjust his medications more rapidly than was possible at home, switching him to a subcutaneous delivery system. Within six hours, his pain was down to an acceptable level, but he was now confused and delirious. He was talking openly about death, referring in sentence fragments to aspects of his past life in ways that the family could not comprehend. He was restless, and could not be comforted. Switching to alternate analgesics did not resolve the problem, nor did the usual antianxiety and antipsychotic medications. Mr. B.'s family members were beside themselves with worry, as the peace and dignity that they had worked so hard to achieve over the past four months seemed to be falling apart. After exhausting all alternatives intended to relieve his agitation and delirium, he was started on a sedating infusion. It took another six hours to settle him down. As soon as his agitation ceased, he died almost immediately.

Mr. B.'s family found his last hours unnerving, undermining much of their feeling of satisfaction at having been there for their father. In spite of our reassurance that they had done a wonderful job (which was genuinely the case), their most vivid memory of his death remains his last hours of help-lessness and agitation. Because their expectations of helping their father achieve a peaceful death were compromised at the end, they felt that they had let him down, and they were at greater risk for problems with bereave-ment. I have met with Mr. B.'s family members many times, exploring their expectations and perceptions about his end-of-life care. I have tried to reas-sure them that they did everything possible for their father, and that his suffering at the end was small compared to the love and caring they experienced together over many months. Unfortunately, their acceptance and healing will take time.

Potential and Limitations of Pain and Symptom Management

Palliative care, when delivered in the context of a comprehensive interdiscipli-nary program such as hospice, can relieve most but not all terminal suffering.[3,4] Most experts agree that approximately 95% of pain can be relieved in a manner that is acceptable to the patient, which is a remarkable record of effectiveness unless you happen to be one of the unrelieved 5%. These claims are more complex than is ordinarily acknowledged, primarily because most patients have an end-of-life trajectory that may span many months or even years, and pain and other physical symptoms fluctuate throughout the course. Symptoms such as pain usually remain manageable throughout the vast majority of a patient's illness. For some, like Mr. B., this record of effectiveness can be threatened when symptoms accelerate in the last days or weeks of life. Just how excep-tional is Mr. B.'s experience? In surveys of hospice patients, from 2% to 35% report their pain as "severe" or "intolerable" during the last week of life.[4-6] In one report, 25% of hospice patients reported their shortness of breath as "unbearable" in the last week of life.[6]

Furthermore, the symptoms that frequently accompany dying are varied, including nausea, vomiting, or open wounds that may be less amenable to expert palliation. The most commonly cited reason for requesting physician-assisted death is not pain, but rather increasing weakness, debility, fatigue, and dependence.[7-10] Many patients with terminal delirium lose the capacity to make decisions for themselves toward the end. When a patient quietly drifts into an increasingly somnolent state resembling a deep sleep owing to the progressive metabolic changes of dying, family members and caregivers may feel reassured that death is coming peacefully. On the other hand, when a patient becomes agitated, like Mr. B., the source of the agitation becomes more complex, often threatening the gratification that might otherwise have come from caring for a loved one. The decision to sedate such a patient, who now can no longer consent to the intervention, is both morally and clinically complex.[11] (This topic will be covered in Chapter 12.) For Mr. B., our efforts to try to preserve his consciousness while relieving his distress meant 48 hours of his talking "out of his mind." Instead of attributing this agitation to the metabolic changes that accompany dying, Mr. B.'s family and some of the hospice staff worried that it might be indicative of "unfinished business" with God or with his family. Unfortunately, they now remember the discomfort and uncertainty of those last hours more vividly than the months when they helped to provide peace, comfort, and a continued presence in his home.

Because many patients and families have seen less than completely peaceful deaths in hospice, we must not over- or under-promise about what we can provide. Certainly expertise in pain and symptom management are cornerstones to good end-of-life care. However, we also need a plan for handling tough symptoms, such as agitated delirium, if they threaten a patient's integrity during the dying process. Those who say "no" to allowing physician-assisted suicide must develop alternative approaches for circumstances where physical symptoms become so severe as to threaten the integrity of the person.[12] Terminal sedation may not be elegant as a "last-resort" response, but it is better than providing no choice. Perhaps the physician's most important commitment is to see the process through with the patient and family, for it is impossible to predict what kind of challenges may arise.[13]

Mr. B. had the best care that hospice has to offer. He was able to spend quality time at home with his family, and during that time his pain and other symptoms were well controlled. He did not like the weakness and dependence that accompanied his disease progression, but he was willing to tolerate them provided he could have more quality time at home with his family. When his symptoms accelerated at the end and agitated terminal delirium developed, the hospice team worked diligently to find a solution. Although it took a few days to adequately control his symptoms, the family, hoping at first to preserve his consciousness but later accepting heavy sedation, had a team of skilled caregivers with whom to work. The patient, his family, and the entire health care team all pursued the same goal of relieving his suffering in a way consistent with Mr. B.'s values and wishes.

The Hospice Philosophy Is Not for Everyone

Two overarching goals are embraced in the hospice movement. The first is to relieve physical suffering by effectively managing pain and any other symptoms that may emerge at any time in the dying process. Relieving such suffering is, of course, a good in itself, yet one of the reasons often cited for achieving this end is so that the patient's personal, emotional, and spiritual energy can be released for the important matters of end-of-life resolution.[14] Thus, the second goal of the hospice movement is to allow the patient and his or her loved ones time to prepare for death: healing emotional wounds with family members, making peace with one's God, and reviewing and passing on important family stories. Developmental tasks that might be undertaken in the dying process include seeking and giving forgiveness for past wrongs, expressing and allowing the expression of love and caring, accepting the increasing dependence that accompanies dying, and allowing family members to "give back" care to the dying person.

This opportunity for personal growth can prove meaningful to dying patients who may have defined themselves in other ways in the past. Many adults express their self-worth and personal identity in terms of work, physical activity, or perhaps taking care of others. Accepting the dependency of terminal illness, and allowing oneself to be the recipient rather than the giver of care, requires an enormous leap of faith. Whereas much may be gained in this transformation, such "growth" is not for everyone. Sometimes it is a matter of timing. For example, when Mr. B. first learned of hospice, he was not ready to "give up" on aggressive therapy, nor was he interested in talking about or accepting his death. He understood the subtext of what I was saying to him (*"You are likely dying no matter what we do, and aggressive treatment may help but more likely will add to your suffering without enhancing your length or quality of life."*). He was not offended or frightened by this seemingly pessimistic information, but he still wanted to keep hospice in reserve for a later time. Even as he was pursuing an aggressive approach to his disease, we emphasized expert pain and symptom management and periodically talked about the importance of a will and of unaddressed spiritual issues "just in case things did not go as we hoped." Mr. B did not want to pursue these issues in depth, yet partly as a result of these discussions he knew that time with his children and grandchildren was growing more precious, and he took full advantage of it. When his symptoms accelerated and it became clear that even experimental therapy was not working, he accepted a hospice referral.

Most of Mr. B.'s existential and spiritual work was nonverbal. He spent time with his family, but talk with them about his dying was rarely explicit. Nevertheless, he *showed* his family how much he loved them, and how much he appreciated their caring, with a smile or a hug or a tear. It was how Mr. B. and his family operated, and it clearly needed to be honored and respected. This would be Mr. B.'s final chapter, and his values and preferences guided the script.

Some patients and families equate giving up on aggressive treatment with giving up on life. They prefer instead to fight their disease to the death, "raging against the darkness," using medical technology as their main weapon. When standard therapies fail, such patients frequently seek experimental therapies. When these treatments fail, they search out physicians or others who are willing to continue to experiment with them in desperate hope of finding something that will suppress their disease. Death is rarely something to be accepted for such patients, but the fight against disease has critical meaning. Such patients may be depriving themselves of the opportunity to accept their inevitable death and formally say good-bye to their families and friends, but they gain the meaning that comes with a heroic medical battle against all odds. Even when patients are engaged in these improbable fights against disease and death, pain and symptoms should be carefully addressed. These elements of palliative care are appropriate for all seriously ill patients, no matter what their prognosis or how invasive their disease-related treatment. In addition, if such patients and their families are willing to explore end-of-life issues "just in case" the battle is not won, this should also be encouraged.

Informed consent for such experimental therapies is an important issue. With regard to experimental therapies, clinicians must be honest with patients and families about the odds of success (very low), the nature of success (usually temporary disease suppression rather than cure), and the kind of increased suffering that may accompany a particular treatment. Patients and their families must be informed about hospice as a reasonable alternative, including the idea that there is nothing about hospice that precludes a "miracle," if that is what the patient or family is looking for. Taking time to think over options is desirable, since the odds of success usually do not change with small delays, and the side effects of experimental therapy are likely to define in large measure the last phase of a patient's life. Once full informed consent is achieved, the patient should be supported in whatever decision is made, and should be permitted a change of heart no matter which treatment is chosen.

Some patients and families choose a hospice approach, but long-standing communication problems and even abuse can be difficult to manage, much less resolve, even with the help of a skilled and committed hospice team. Working with such families is challenging for hospice caregivers who believe it is part of their mission to help families achieve some level of forgiveness and acceptance before a loved one's death. With the expertise, encouragement, and support of hospice team members, sometimes forgiveness and healing can be achieved even in seemingly difficult families. Other patients and families may see these issues as dangerous or uncomfortable to deal with, and choose not to work on or even discuss them. The challenge of this aspect of hospice care is to give patients the opportunity to work on these issues, perhaps even encourage them to do so, but ultimately to accept the decision of the patient and family in this matter.

Prognostic Uncertainty and Hospice Program Requirements

To be eligible for the Medicare hospice benefit, a patient must be "terminally ill," which is defined as having a prognosis of six months or less. On the surface, this time frame might seem like a reasonable public policy requirement. Hospice programs were originally designed for cancer patients, and there was a common belief that all cancers followed a predictable time course. However, only about one-third of deaths in the United States are from cancer, and not all cancers follow this kind of trajectory. Prostate cancer, the cancer that Mr. B had, is a case in point. Some prostate cancers are very aggressive, and once they fail to be controlled, death may well come within the six-month hospice guideline. Other prostate cancers, particularly in the elderly, tend to be more indolent, and patients can live for years with widespread disease.

Suppose a patient with a quality of life he describes as "poor" wanted treatment devoted only to his comfort and dignity, and to use his remaining time to bring resolution to his life. Perhaps his odds of dying in six months are 50%, but his odds of living two years are 25%. From a philosophical and clinical vantage point, he would be an ideal candidate for hospice, but he would not qualify because we are not sure enough that he would die in the prescribed time frame.

The majority of deaths in this country come not from cancer, but rather from some combination of advanced cardiac, pulmonary, neurological, and renal diseases.[15] Most patients with advanced stages of congestive heart failure, chronic obstructive lung disease, or dementia do not qualify for hospice, even if they choose to forgo aggressive treatment of their underlying diseases and seek to maximize their comfort and dignity in their remaining time. Many patients in my practice have let it be known through their advance directives that should they develop Alzheimer's disease in the future, they want comfort measures only. They want to forgo disease-related treatment, even of infections or other reversible problems. Such patients would be ideal hospice candidates both clinically and philosophically. Yet the nature of their disease does not allow for a terminal prognosis with any degree of certainty, so they do not qualify for Medicare-sponsored hospice services. Their symptoms can still be managed aggressively to maximize comfort, and the patients can be protected from cardiopulmonary resuscitation by completing a do-not-resuscitate document, but there are no comprehensive palliative care programs like hospice to help them find the most meaning possible in the time that remains to them.

A few innovative programs in this country receive Medicare waivers to provide hospice-type care for patients with dementia.[16] More frequently, such patients are "treated" in the traditional medical system rather than "cared for," and are repeatedly admitted to an acute hospital setting for intervening complications such as infections or eating problems. The goals of treatment (though usually not explicitly stated) emphasize life prolongation and ignore associated human suffering, with little consideration of the patient's values and prestated wishes. Such disease-driven, aggressive medical intervention often seems harsh and purposeless, and clearly it needs to be redressed if we are to create a humane health care system for patients with dementia.

Similarly, some patients with advanced congestive heart failure have decided not to receive cardiopulmonary resuscitation in the future, but rather treatment geared toward maximizing their comfort and dignity. Such patients may want to minimize but not completely eliminate intravenous treatments, blood tests, or X rays. If they develop severe shortness of breath in the future, they may want a trial of increased diuretics, but if they fail to respond, they may want to be sedated rather than put on a mechanical ventilator. Many of these patients have been in and out of the hospital frequently, and many know and even accept that they are near death. Some would welcome the opportunity to work on issues of life closure, and would benefit greatly from a hospice program, but do not meet the prognostic requirements for Medicare. A patient with advanced congestive heart failure has a 50% chance of living six months on the day before he or she dies, and a 25% chance of living one year.[17] They therefore would be systematically excluded from Medicare-sponsored hospice programs based on prognosis, unless they chose to stop all their medications and were near death.[18]

Hospice programs would be ideally suited for many patients with less certain terminal prognoses, but, as currently constructed, the hospice Medicare benefit may be too personnel and resource intensive to be offered to them. Estimates of cost savings derived from hospice care are somewhat controversial, but it is clear that most of the savings as compared to traditional care appear to be achieved in the last few months of life.[19] Hospice programs tend to break even at about six months of survival as compared to traditional care, and become more costly when patients survive for nine to 12 months or more.[19] The cost savings derived from preventing unwanted cardiopulmonary resuscitation or long unwanted stays in intensive care are hard to estimate, but they must be substantial. Such stays are not only costly, but they are demoralizing to families and medical personnel, who can lose a sense of purpose when medicine seems only to be prolonging suffering and dying.

Disease-Related Treatment and Palliative Care

A second requirement of the Medicare hospice benefit is that patients forgo aggressive disease-related treatment. Again, using the cancer model, this would include intensive chemotherapy or radiotherapy directed at cure or at long-term remission. Such treatments are very expensive, and hospice is reimbursed at a fixed amount each day (about $100), which must cover all medical expenses, including medications. Not only is such aggressive treatment likely to engender considerable additional suffering, but it is very expensive and could easily bankrupt a program if repeatedly offered. Chemotherapy, radiation, or surgery directed at palliating an uncomfortable symptom (for example, a painful local area of bony involvement) would be allowed as part of the Medicare hospice benefit, since its purpose is symptom management and not disease treatment.

Even within the realm of cancer treatment, certain inexpensive disease-related treatments might be continued after enrollment in a hospice program. For example, hormone treatment of prostate or breast cancer that is suppressing the disease could be continued as long as the patient's quality of life warranted it. In addition, pulmonary or kidney infections might be treated early during a hospice stay, provided the patient's wishes and quality of life call for it, whereas later, as death approaches, these treatments might be discontinued or not started. In the area of noncancer diseases, such choices and trade-offs are more commonplace and more complex.

Mrs. M. was a 90 year-old woman with pulmonary fibrosis and congestive heart failure. She had been hospitalized three times in the last year for pneumonia, and had made a decision to forgo cardiopulmonary resuscitation and mechanical ventilation but to try any and all noninvasive measures to prolong her life. However, Mrs. M.'s last hospitalization was long and traumatic, and she vowed never to return to the hospital. She would stay home, even if septic, and try oral antibiotics. Despite this decision, Mrs. M. did not qualify for a hospice program, based on her prognosis and the fact that she wanted to continue her many medications and have a trial of noninvasive treatment for future infections. Whether and how we could support her at home without the assistance of a hospice team if she developed severe breathing problems was highly problematic.

Four months later, she developed shaking chills and a large lower-lobe pneumonia. She began vomiting, and could not keep her medications down. She said she would rather die than go back to the hospital, but she was not prepared to die if her disease could be treated relatively easily. I convinced her to be admitted to our inpatient palliative care unit, where we would treat her with intravenous antibiotics and fluids but minimize all invasive testing and intervention. I promised that if the suffering was unacceptable to her, we would stop all treatment and provide sedation. I would help to arrange for her to die at home if she deteriorated and wished to be discharged. Fortunately (and somewhat surprisingly), she responded within two days to the intravenous antibiotics and fluids, and she went home in five days feeling considerably better. Mrs. M. has a relatively good quality of life, living independently with the support of her daughter.

Mrs. M. has had excellent symptom management, and is prepared to die when her time comes. She has a home do-not-resuscitate document, and an advance directive stating that all treatments should be discontinued should she lose the capacity to make decisions for herself. She has completed her will, and she is at peace with her God and her family. She knows that she could die any day, and she is prepared. She is an ideal hospice patient, except that her wish to continue noninvasive life-sustaining therapy and her uncertain prognosis disqualify her for hospice care. She remains alive with a reasonably good quality of life one year after her last hospitalization.

Hospice-like programs are ideal for patients, like Mrs. M., who want to forgo invasive, expensive, high-technology treatments but still want to continue disease-related treatments as long as their quality of life remains acceptable.[15] Such patients want and deserve both palliative care and basic disease-related care; nothing about these approaches should make them mutually exclusive. Perhaps such programs cannot be as resource intensive as current hospice programs are, but they must include pain and symptom management, advance care planning, and some opportunity to work on issues of life closure if the patient wishes. Such programs should be developed for all patients with a significant disease burden who have a strong likelihood of dying in 6 to 12 months. Combined palliative care and disease-management programs might be developed for nursing home patients and those with advanced congestive heart failure, chronic lung disease, kidney failure, and dementia, for example. As long as patients can continue any disease-directed treatment that they choose, there is no reason to exclude them from approaches that can enhance both the quality of their lives and the quality of their deaths. Many innovative programs are currently seeking Medicare waivers to provide this type of care.

Palliative Care, Hospice, and Physician-Assisted Death

The National Hospice Organization and the AMA have taken firm positions against the legalization of physician-assisted suicide,[20,21] yet physicians in general, like the general population, are divided on this issue, with more in favor than against.[22-26] Surveys are frequently limited by the framing bias of the questioners. When the question "Would you rather have access to hospice or to a physician-assisted death?" is posed, most of us would answer in favor of hospice. On the other hand, if the question is reframed as "If your dying becomes intolerable to you in spite of excellent hospice care, would you want access to a physician-assisted death as a last resort?" the percent favoring open access to physician-assisted death would likely be much higher.

Hospice care is the standard of care for the dying against which any other treatment or intervention must be measured. In spite of the promise of hospice, some patients—like Diane (Chapter 3)—fear future suffering, dependence, and lack of control of mind and body. They need to know that there will be an escape from their worst-case scenario in order to have the peace of mind and spirit to make the most of their time remaining. Diane lived for three months supported by a hospice program once she knew she could end her life if her suffering became unacceptable. She had excellent pain and symptom management, and she took several life-prolonging treatments for infections in that time because her quality of life was good and her "business" with family and friends was not yet finished. Diane grew much closer to her husband and son during that three-month period; hospice nurses commented that she was the kind of open and articulate person who drew them to hospice work in the first place.

Most people who, like Diane, fear future suffering will be reassured by the possibility of an escape if their suffering becomes unacceptable to them. The escape need not be physician-assisted suicide. For some, it is the assurance of potentially sedating doses of pain medication if they are dying in severe pain, and for others it is the promise of heavy sedation if they become "out of their mind" with delirium. Since Diane was fearful about losing control of her body and mind, the prospect of strong sedatives was not reassuring to her compared to having access to potentially lethal medication. Many patients are reassured by the possibility of terminal sedation as a last resort, so Diane was the exception and not the rule. Of course, we have to care for exceptions as well as rules, so we must be as creative and innovative as possible.

Some patients, like both Mr. B. and Diane, reach a point where their suffering becomes intolerable and they need an escape. For Diane, it was increasing pain accompanied by sepsis. Her life without taking the overdose would have lasted a few days to at most a week, but that time of rapidly accelerating disability and suffering would have been her worst nightmare. She received and took advantage of the best hospice had to offer. In her estimation, for her to take an overdose at the very end was not inconsistent with the hospice philosophy. Up to that point, she had had excellent pain and symptom management, had done the psychological and spiritual work of life resolution, and had accepted her death as inevitable. Her death at that moment was a fitting escape after making the most of the time she had.

Similarly, Mr. B. had an excellent experience in hospice, received excellent pain and symptom management, and achieved closure with his family on his own terms. At the very end, he needed an escape from escalating pain and then mental agitation that could be achieved only with complete sedation. His family's only regret was that we did not sedate him more quickly than we did.

Most patients do not want to make a choice between access to hospice and access to a physician-assisted death. Instead, they want access to excellent palliative care services no matter how uncertain their prognosis, even if they choose to continue some or all of their disease-related treatments. They also want us to assure them that we will remain responsive if their suffering becomes intolerable in spite of excellent care. We must respond effectively and forthrightly to those rare patients who experience severe symptoms prior to death, for they and their families are counting on us to be unafraid. The challenge in these troubling situations is to find the least objectionable way to respond given the patient's clinical situation, values, and wishes, and the values of the family and immediate health care providers.[27] Those who say "no" to physician-assisted suicide must develop a way of approaching these tough cases; terminal sedation is one potential way. All responses of last resort are imperfect, yet they are better than abandoning the patient and family to extremes of suffering or acting on their own in secret.

References

1. Cancer Pain Relief and Palliative Care. Technical Report Series 804. 1990. Geneva: World Health Organization.
2. Stoddard S. Hospice in the United States: An overview. *J Palliat Care* 1989; 5:10.
3. Wallston KA, Burger C, Smith RA, Baugher RJ. Comparing the quality of death for hospice and non-hospice cancer patients. *Med Care* 1988; 26:177–182.
4. Kasting GA. The nonnecessity of euthanasia. In: Humber JD, Almeder RF, Kasting GA, editors. *Physician-Assisted Death*. Totawa, NJ: Humana Press, 1993, pp. 25–43.
5. Ventafridda V, Ripamonti C, DeConno F, Tamburini M, Cassileth BR. Symptom prevalence and control during cancer patients' last days of life. *J Palliat Care* 1990; 6:7–11.
6. Coyle N, Adelhardt J, Foley KM, Portenoy RK. Character of terminal illness in the advanced cancer patient: Pain and other symptoms during the last four weeks of life. *J Pain Symptom Manage* 1990; 5:83–93.

7. American Board of Internal Medicine Committee. Caring for the Dying: Identification and Promotion of Physician Competency. 1–100. 1996. Philadelphia, American Board of Internal Medicine.

8. van der Maas PJ, van der Wal G, Haverkate I, de Graaff CL, Kester JG, Onwuteaka-Philipsen BD, et al. Euthanasia, physician-assisted suicide, and other medical practices involving the end of life in the Netherlands, 1990–1995. *N Engl J Med* 1996; 335:1699–1705.

9. Back AL, Wallace JI, Starks HE, Pearlman RA. Physician-assisted suicide and euthanasia in Washington State: Patient requests and physician responses. *JAMA* 1996; 275:919–925.

10. Chin AE, Hedberg K, Higginson GK, Fleming DW. Legalized physician-assisted suicide in Oregon—the first year's experience. *N Engl J Med* 1999; 340(7):577–583.

11. Quill TE, Lo, Brock DW. Palliative options of last resort: A comparison of voluntarily stopping eating and drinking, terminal sedation, physician-assisted suicide, and voluntary active euthanasia. *JAMA* 1997; 278:1099–2104.

12. Quill TE, Byock I. Responding to intractable terminal suffering: the role of terminal sedation and voluntary refusal of food and fluids. ACP-ASIM End-of-Life Care Consensus Panel. *Ann Intern Med* 2000; 132:408–414.

13. Quill TE, Cassel CK. Nonabandonment: A central obligation for physicians. *Ann Intern Med* 1995; 122:368–374.

14. Byock I. *Dying Well: The Prospect for Growth at the End of Life.* New York: Riverhead Books, 1997.

15. Wanzer SH, Federman DD, Adelstein SJ, Cassel CK, Cassem EH, Cranford RE, et al. The physician's responsibility toward hopelessly ill patients: A second look. *N Engl J Med* 1989; 320:844–849.

16. Volicer L, Rheaume Y, Brown J, Fabiscewski K, Brady R. Hospice approach to the treatment of patients with advanced dementia of the Alzheimer type. *JAMA* 1986; 256:2210–2213.

17. Lynn J, Harrell F Jr, Cohn F, Wagner D, Connors AF Jr. Prognoses of seriously ill hospitalized patients on the days before death: Implications for patient care and public policy. *New Horizons* 1997; 5(1):56–61.

18. Morita T, Tsunoda J, Inoue S, Chihara S. The Palliative Prognostic Index: A scoring system for survival prediction of terminally ill cancer patients. *Supportive Care in Cancer* 1999; 7(3):128–133128.

19. Emanuel EJ, Battin MP. What are the potential cost savings from legalizing physician-assisted suicide? *N Engl J Med* 1998; 339:167–172.

20. National Hospice Organization. (1990). Statement of the National Hospice Organization Opposing the Legalization of Euthanasia and Assisted Suicide.

21. American Medical Association. Report of the Council on Ethical and Judicial Affairs of the American Medical Association on Physician-Assisted Suicide. *Issues Law Med* 1994; 10:91–97.

22. Shapiro R, Derse AR, Gottlieb M, Scheidermayer D, Olson M. Willingness to perform euthanasia: A survey of physician attitudes. *Arch Intern Med* 1994; 154:575–584.

23. Lee MA, Nelson HD, Tilden VP, Ganzini L, Schmidt TA, Tolle SW. Legalizing assisted suicide—views of physicians in Oregon. *N Engl J Med* 1996; 334:310–315.

24. Duberstein PR, Conwell Y, Cox C, Podgorski CA, Glazer RS, Caine ED. Attitudes toward self-determined death: A survey of primary care physicians. *J Am Geriatr Soc* 1995; 43:395–400.

25. Cohen JS, Fihn SD, Boyko EJ, Jonsen AR, Wood RW. Attitudes toward assisted suicide and euthanasia among physicains in Washington State. *N Engl J Med* 1994; 331:89–94.
26. Emanuel EJ, Fairclough DL, Daniels ER, Clarridge BR. Euthanasia and physician-assisted suicide: attitudes and experiences of oncology patients, oncologists, and the public. *Lancet* 1996; 347:1805–1810.
27. Quill TE, Coombs-Lee B, Nunn S. Palliative options of last resort: Choosing the least harmful alternative. *Ann Intern Med* 2000; 132:488–493.

11

The Rule of Double Effect: A Critique of Its Role in End-of-Life Decision Making

According to the ethical principle known as the "rule of double effect," effects that would be morally wrong if caused intentionally are permissible if foreseen but unintended. This principle is often cited to explain why certain forms of care at the end of life that result in death are morally permissible and others are not.[1-9] According to this rule, administering high-dose opioids to lessen a terminally ill patient's pain may be acceptable even if the medication causes the patient's death. In contrast, it does not authorize practices such as physician-assisted suicide, voluntary euthanasia, and certain instances of forgoing life-sustaining treatment.

The rule of double effect is a conceptually and psychologically complex doctrine that distinguishes between permissible and prohibited actions by relying heavily on the clinician's intent. The doctrine's complexities and ambiguities have limited its value as a guide to clinical practice.[10] This chapter examines the rule's religious and philosophical origins, its inconsistencies with current law, and its shortcomings as a practical clinical guide. Alternative principles are also proposed.

An earlier version of this chapter was co-authored with Rebecca Dresser and Dan Brock, and published in the *New England Journal of Medicine* 1997; 337:1768–1771. I am solely responsible for the added material and editing.

Background

The rule of double effect, which was developed by Roman Catholic moral theologians in the Middle Ages[11,12] is applied to situations in which it is impossible for a person to avoid causing some harm.[11-15] In such situations, a person must decide whether one potentially harmful action is preferable to another.

Suppose a terminally ill man experiencing unrelenting pain and suffering asks his physician for help in ending his misery. If the physician kills the patient to end the patient's suffering, his death is intended. According to the rule of double effect, the goal of relieving the patient's pain and suffering is good, but the means chosen to achieve the goal is wrong. Our moral system prohibits the intentional killing of innocent persons.[11,12]

The word "intentional" suggests, however, that deaths of innocent persons may be permissible if brought about unintentionally. With the same goal of relieving this patient's unbearable pain and suffering, the physician could provide large doses of analgesic medication, even though the patient may die sooner as a result. If the physician refrains from providing such medication because of the lethal risk it poses, his failure to intervene harms the patient by allowing potentially treatable pain to continue. However, if he provides the medication, it may hasten the patient's death and thus inflict a different harm. The rule of double effect construes the physician's provision of medication in the second scenario as an intentional action to relieve pain and suffering with the foreseen but unintended risk of causing an earlier death. The physician's action thus does not violate the prohibition against intentionally killing innocent persons.

Classic formulations of the rule of double effect emphasize four key conditions[15] which are summarized in Table 11–1.[16,17] The first concerns the nature of the act itself. It must be good (such as to relieve pain), or at least morally neutral, and not in a category that is absolutely prohibited (such as the killing of innocent persons). The second concerns the agent's intent in performing an act. The "good effect and not the evil effect must be intended." The "evil" effect, such as respiratory depression after administering opioids, may be "foreseen, but not intended." The third condition involves distinguishing between means and effects. The bad effect, such as death, must not be a means to the good effect, such as the relief of suffering. The fourth condition is the proportionality between the good effect and the bad effect. The good effect must outweigh the bad effect. The bad effect can be permitted only when there is "proportionally grave reason" for it.

The first condition is used to determine whether an act is ever potentially permissible; the second and third conditions are used to determine whether the potential harm that results is intentional or unintentional, as either a means

TABLE 11–1. The Rule of Double Effect: Four Key Elements

1. The act must be good or at least morally neutral.
2. The agent must intend the good effect and not the evil effect (which may be "foreseen" but not intended).
3. The evil effect must not be the means to the good effect.
4. There must be a "proportionately grave reason" to risk the evil effect.

or an end. The fourth condition requires the agent to compare the net good and bad effects of potentially acceptable actions to determine which course would produce an effect of proportionately greater value. Thus, the agent should choose the action with the most favorable balance of good and bad effects, within the limits set by the first three conditions of the rule.

Clinical Applications of the Rule of Double Effect to End-of-Life Decisions

Recall Mr. B., the man with metastatic prostate cancer who was presented at the beginning of Chapter 10. With respect to the opioids and sedatives used to treat his pain and suffering, the rule of double effect might have been considered at three points in his illness:

1. When Mr. B first had pain, and was reluctant about taking opioids, his fears were that he would become "addicted" or that the medication would lose its effectiveness if used over a long period of time. He was able to be reassured on both accounts, and began taking the medication with significant improvement of his pain. At that time, neither he nor I, as his physician, was afraid of his dying prematurely as an unintended consequence of the opioids, nor was there a significant risk of his doing so.[18] In fact, there are some preliminary data that suggest patients with adequate pain relief tend to live longer, and certainly their quality of life is improved. If Mr. B. had a rare, idiosyncratic lethal side effect to the medication, then death could in no way have been intended or anticipated by the clinician, and there would be no need to invoke the rule of double effect.

2. Later, when Mr. B. was more actively dying and his pain was rapidly increasing in intensity, the risk of accelerating death because of the need for rapidly escalating doses of opioids was real. Neither Mr. B. nor I, as his physician, was intending to hasten his death, but the severity of his pain and suffering along with the nearness of his inevitable death made

the need to take the risk (of sedating him or causing some respiratory depression, and thereby hastening death) compelling. Mr. B., his family, and I were all very conscious of this risk, and could foresee that this could happen as an unwanted and unintended side effect, but it in no way was the purpose of the treatment. His suffering was proportionate enough to warrant the risk, so therefore this action met all criteria for the rule of double effect.

3. When Mr. B. became delirious from the combined metabolic effects of his dying and the side effects of his analgesic treatments, we had a more complex dilemma. Allowing him to remain agitated when we could provide relief by sedating him would have been unacceptable. Clearly the severity of his suffering and the nearness of his inevitable death warranted taking a substantial risk of hastening death as a potential side effect, especially if there were no less harmful alternatives. Mr. B.'s intent was to escape from his suffering, and he was willing to accept that death might come earlier as an unintended consequence of our action. If the sedating medication relieved his agitation without rendering him unconscious, we would not have further increased the dose. Similarly, we did not increase the dose once he appeared comfortably sedated. This, then, would seem to fall within the purview of the rule of double effect. However, we still had to address the question of whether to continue intravenous fluids, because while Mr. B. was sedated he had no way to eat or drink. Our intent in withholding life supports is less simply addressed within the rule of double effect. He is now free from acute suffering, and life support would prolong his life. Although he is legally within his rights to not start such life-sustaining therapy, the condition that has made the treatment necessary is iatrogenic. The physician's and the patient's intent in withholding life supports is more problematic for the rule of double effect, making the aggregate act (sedating and withholding treatment) questionable for those who believe in this doctrine.

The rule of double effect is not necessary or relevant for usual pain treatment, as in circumstance 1 above, since the risk of hastening death is no different from many other treatments where the rule is not invoked. In the second circumstance, the rule can help explain why a clinician is permitted to administer very high doses of opioid analgesics to relieve severe pain in a terminally ill patient toward the end of life, even in amounts that could cause the patient to die sooner than he or she would otherwise.[1-9] The physician's goal in these circumstances is to relieve the patient's suffering. The means are the use of opioid analgesics in doses that might contribute to an earlier death. Neither the patient nor the physician intends for the patient to die, either as a means or as

an end. If death occurs, it is an unintended (though in this case possibly foreseen) side effect. The more severe and intractable the patient's pain, the greater
the justification for risking an earlier death. Thus, the amount of opioid pain
reliever that is given and the rapidity with which it is increased must be in
proportion to the patient's pain and suffering.

Some physicians have been reluctant to use sufficient doses of opioid
pain relievers even when their patients are dying, in part because of fears
(both ethical and legal) of contributing to an earlier death.[19] The rule of double
effect has helped some physicians to overcome this hesitation. However, other
clinicians remain unwilling to prescribe sufficient doses because they do not
distinguish morally or psychologically between actions performed with the
intent to cause death and those performed with the foreseen possibility of
causing death.[7,20,21]

The rule of double effect is also of limited assistance in evaluating the practice of terminal sedation described in circumstance 3 above.[22–25] In this situation, the consenting patient is sedated to the point of unconsciousness in order
to relieve otherwise untreatable pain and suffering, and is then allowed to die
of dehydration or other intervening complications. The goal of administering
the sedative, to relieve otherwise unrelievable suffering, is good. Whether death
is intended or merely foreseen is less clear. Unlike the use of high-dose opioids
to relieve pain, with death as a possible but undesired side effect, terminal sedation inevitably causes death. In many cases, as with the physician and patient
in the previous chapter, death as a means to escape suffering is what the patient
desires. Although the overall goal of terminal sedation is to relieve otherwise
uncontrollable suffering, life-prolonging therapies are withdrawn with the
intent of hastening death. Terminal sedation would thus be problematic under
the rule of double effect, even though it is usually considered acceptable
according to current legal and medical ethical standards.[25–27]

Voluntary euthanasia, in which the physician knowingly and intentionally
administers a lethal injection at the request of a suffering patient, clearly
violates the rule's requirement that death not be intentionally caused as a means
or an end.[22] An analysis of physician-assisted suicide, where the physician knowingly provides a terminally ill suffering patient with medication that could be
used as a lethal overdose, is more complex. The goal of physician-assisted
suicide is to relieve intolerable suffering, but the means to this end are to
provide the patient with a potential death-producing agent.[22] Providing a
patient with a means to end life could be held to violate the prohibition against
intentionally causing death (or contributing to the patient's intentional act of
ending his or her own life), even if the physician's overarching purpose is to
relieve intolerable suffering. Yet the physician may have many purposes in providing such prescriptions:[10,28] to offer a sleeping aid; to reassure the patient by
providing a potential escape from suffering that the physician hopes or expects

will not be used; or to relieve suffering, with death as an inevitable but unintended side effect. The simple classifications of intent provided by the rule of double effect are not easily applied to the physician's intentions in this clinical setting. Moreover, it is the patient's action, not the physician's, that directly causes death in the case of physician-assisted suicide.

Finally, although there is clinical, ethical, and legal consensus that patients have the right to refuse life-sustaining treatment, such decisions are sometimes problematic when analyzed according to the rule of double effect. Some patients with conditions such as advanced emphysema may decide to discontinue mechanical ventilation, knowing they may die but hoping they will be able to live unencumbered by medical technology.[29] In such cases, the clinician is permitted to remove the ventilator under the rule of double effect. Other patients, however, may make the same decision with the explicit intent to escape severe suffering by hastening death.[29,30] In these cases, the rule of double effect might not permit the clinician to remove the ventilator provided he has knowledge of the patient's intention to cause death. The rule may cause confusion about physicians' responsibilities with regard to stopping life support and may account for the reluctance of some physicians to carry out patients' wishes to forgo treatment.[19,31] Some clinicians do not see the rule as an absolute guide to end-of-life decision making. In one large clinical study, 39% of physicians who had sedated patients while stopping life support reported that they had done so with the intention of hastening death, in clear violation of the rule of double effect.[32]

The Rule of Double Effect and U.S. Criminal Law

Recent Supreme Court rulings on physician-assisted suicide illustrate the similarities and differences in how current law and the rule of double effect evaluate a clinician's conduct in various end-of-life circumstances.[26,27] The law incorporates singular considerations in evaluating the administration of pain-relieving opioids. Although criminal law does not exempt from liability all persons who unintentionally cause another person's death, conduct posing a risk to life is permissible if it is justified by the expected benefits. One example is risky surgery performed to correct a serious medical condition.[33] Because the law includes a principle resembling the proportionality provision in the rule of double effect, clinicians may administer potentially lethal medications when they are necessary to relieve a terminally ill patient's suffering.[34]

On the other hand, the rule of double effect and criminal law have different implications with respect to forgoing life-sustaining treatment. In contrast to the rule of double effect, the law permits, indeed requires, clinicians to forgo treatment at the request of a competent patient, even when the express purpose is to cause the patient's death. Similarly, terminal sedation with the patient's informed consent is legally permissible. These practices are lawful because death results from omitting medical interventions refused by patients who are exercising their rights to self-determination and protection of their physical integrity.

Current law joins the rule of double effect in prohibiting clinicians from providing or administering lethal medications with the explicit purpose of causing a patient's death. Here one could argue that the law shares some of the rule's weaknesses and uncertainties. As noted earlier, physicians may have various aims when they provide terminally ill patients with prescriptions for potentially lethal medications. In the case of a patient who ingests a lethal overdose of a drug prescribed by a physician, prosecutors ordinarily would have great difficulty establishing beyond a reasonable doubt that the physician acted intentionally or knowingly to help the patient die, which would be necessary to support a conviction for assisting in suicide. Moreover, the general refusal of jurors to convict physicians charged with assisted suicide or with contributing to the consensual deaths of their suffering, terminally ill patients indicates that many ordinary persons disagree with the prohibition against all intentional direct killing, incorporated in both the rule of double effect and current criminal law.

Ethical and Policy Issues

The rule of double effect has many shortcomings as an ethical guide for either clinical practice or public policy. First, the rule originated in the context of a particular religious tradition.[12,13] American society incorporates multiple religious, ethical, and professional traditions, so medicine must accommodate various approaches to assessing the morality of end-of-life practices. Many persons and groups reject the position that death should never be intentionally hastened when unrelievable suffering is extreme and death is desired by the patient.[35–37] Yet the rule's absolute prohibition against deliberately taking human life seems to apply even to a competent, terminally ill patient who seeks to end suffering through the cessation of life-sustaining therapy.

The analysis of intention used in the rule of double effect is both difficult to validate externally and inconsistent with other analyses of human intention. Even philosophers and theologians sympathetic to the distinction between intended and foreseen consequences have failed to find an unambiguous way to draw the distinction in many difficult cases.[38–40] Moreover, according to modern psychology, human intention is multi-layered, ambiguous, subjective, and often contradictory.[10,41] The rule of double effect does not acknowledge this complexity; instead, intention is judged according to the presence or absence of a clear purpose. Clinicians familiar with the requirements of the rule may learn to express their intentions by performing ambiguous acts such as providing terminal sedation or withdrawing life support with foreseen but unintended consequences; at the same time, other clinicians may reasonably interpret these acts as clear violations of the rule.

In most moral, social, and legal realms, people are held responsible for all reasonably foreseeable consequences of their actions, not just the intended consequences. Physicians are not exempt from this expectation. This understanding of moral responsibility encourages people to exercise due care in their actions and holds them responsible for that which is under their control.[41] The important moral question is whether the risk of foreseeable harm is justified by an action's good effects. It is the principle of proportionality that determines when the risk of undesirable consequences is justified.

Autonomy is a central tenet of Western medical ethics and law.[42,43] Those who give considerable weight to patients' rights to determine their own care believe that a patient's informed consent to an action that may cause death is more fundamental than whether the physician intends to hasten death. From this perspective, the crucial moral considerations in evaluating any act that could cause death are the patient's right to self-determination and bodily integrity, the provision of informed consent, the absence of less harmful alternatives, and the severity of the patient's suffering.

Finally, the rule of double effect has had both desirable and undesirable effects on clinical conduct. The rule has reassured clinicians that prescribing high-dose opioids for pain in terminally ill patients is morally permissible, and that is all to the good.[7] More controversially, the rule has reinforced absolute societal and professional prohibitions against directly and intentionally causing death.[8,9] It also has negative effects on clinical practice, particularly when patients are making decisions that include death as a likely consequence. Concern about violating the rule's absolute prohibition against intentionally causing death may account for the reluctance of some physicians to honor their patients' requests to withdraw life-sustaining therapy.[19,31] Furthermore, the unwillingness of some physicians to provide adequate medication for pain relief, particularly if a medication can contribute to an earlier death, may reflect their failure to accept the rule's simplistic account of intention in such situations.

Concluding Thoughts

For clinicians and others who believe in an absolute prohibition against actions that intentionally cause death, the rule of double effect may be useful as a way of justifying pain relief and other palliative measures for dying patients. But the rule is not a necessary means to that important end. Furthermore, the rule's absolute prohibitions, unrealistic characterization of physicians' intentions, and failure to account for patients' wishes make it problematic in many circumstances. In keeping with the traditions of medicine and broader society, we believe that physicians' care of their dying patients is properly guided and justified by patients' informed consent, the degree of suffering, and the absence of less harmful alternatives to the treatment contemplated.

References

1. American Medical Association's Council on Ethical and Judicial Affairs. Decisions near the end of life. *JAMA* 1992; 276:2229–2233.
2. American Board of Internal Medicine Committee. (1996). *Caring for the Dying: Identification and Promotion of Physician Competency.* 1–100. Philadelphia: American Board of Internal Medicine.
3. American College of Physicians. American College of Physicians' Ethics Manual. *Ann Intern Med* 1992; 3rd(117):947–960.
4. Council on Scientific Affairs AMA. Good care of the dying patient. *JAMA* 1996; 275:474–478.
5. President's Commission for the Study of Ethical Problems in Medicine and Biomedical and Behavioral Research. (1983). Deciding to forgo life-sustaining treatment: A report on the ethical, medical and legal issues in treatment decisions. Washington, DC: United States Government Printing Office.
6. Hastings Center. *Guidelines on the Termination of Life-Sustaining Treatment and the Care of the Dying.* 1987. New York: The Hastings Center.
7. Foley KM. Competent care for the dying instead of physician-assisted suicide. *N Engl J Med* 1997; 336:54–58.
8. Pellegrino ED. Doctors must not kill. *J Clin Ethics* 1992; 3:95–102.
9. Kass LR. Is there a right to die? *Hastings Cent Rep* 1993; January/February:89–94.
10. Quill TE. The ambiguity of clinical intentions. *N Engl J Med* 1993; 329:1039–1040.
11. The history of intention in ethics. In: Kenny AJP, editor. *Anatomy of the Soul.* Oxford, England: Basil Blackwell, 1973.
12. Mangan JT. An historical analysis of the principle of double effect. *Theol Studies* 1949; 10:41–61.
13. *Evangelium Vitae.* 95 A.D.; Washington, D.C.: U.S. Catholic Conference, 1995.
14. Granfield D. *The Abortion Decision.* Garden City, NY: Image Books, 1971.
15. Garcia JLA. Double effect. In: Reich WT, editor. *Encyclopedia of Bioethics.* New York: Simon and Schuster, 1995: 636–641.
16. Marquis DB. Four versions of the double effect. *J Med Philos* 1991; 16:515–544.
17. Kuhse H. *The Sanctity-of-Life Doctrine in Medicine: A Critique.* Oxford, England: Clarenden Press, 1987.
18. Fohr SA. The double effect of pain medication: Separating myth from reality. *J Palliat Med* 1998; 1:315–328.
19. Solomon MZ, O'Donnell L, Jennings B, Guilfoy V, Wolf SM, Nolan K, et al. Decisions near the end of life: Professional views on life-sustaining treatments. *Am J Public Health* 1993; 83:14–23.

20. Foley KM. Pain, physician-assisted suicide, and euthanasia. *Pain Forum* 1995; 4:163–178.
21. Hill CS Jr. When will adequate pain treatment be the norm? *JAMA* 1995; 274:1881–1882.
22. Quill TE, Lo B, Brock DW. Palliative options of last resort: A comparison of voluntarily stopping eating and drinking, terminal sedation, physician-assisted suicide, and voluntary active euthanasia. *JAMA* 1997; 278:1099–2104.
23. Troug RD, Berde DB, Mitchell C, Grier HE. Barbiturates in the care of the terminally ill. *N Engl J Med* 1991; 327:1678–1682.
24. Ventafridda V, Ripamonti C, DeConno F, Tamburini M, Cassileth BR. Symptom prevalence and control during cancer patients' last days of life. *J Palliat Care* 1990; 6:7–11.
25. Cherny NI, Portenoy RK. Sedation in the management of refractory symptoms: Guidelines for evaluation and treatment. *J Palliat Care* 1994; 10:31–38.
26. *Vacco v. Quill.* 1997. 117 S.Ct. 2293.
27. *Washington v. Glucksberg.* 1997. 117 S.Ct 2258.
28. Annas GJ. The promised end—constitutional aspects of physician-assisted suicide. *N Engl J Med* 1996; 335:683–687.
29. Alpers A, Lo B. Does it make clinical sense to equate terminally ill patients who require life-sustaining interventions with those who do not? *JAMA* 1997; 277:1705–1708.
30. Orentlicher D. The legalization of physician-assisted suicide. *N Engl J Med* 1996; 335:663–667.
31. The SUPPORT Principal Investigators. A controlled trial to improve care for seriously ill hospitalized patients. The study to understand prognoses and preferences for outcomes and risks of treatment (SUPPORT). *JAMA* 1995; 274:591–1598.
32. Wilson WC, Smedira NG, Fink C, McDowell JA, Luce JM. Ordering and administration of sedatives and analgesics during the withholding and withdrawal of life support from critically ill patients. *JAMA* 1992; 267:949–953.
33. American Law Institute. *Model Penal Code and Commentaries*. Section 2.02 ed. Philadelphia: American Law Institute, 1985.
34. Cantor NL, Thomas GC. Pain relief, acceleration of death, and criminal law. *Kennedy Inst Ethics J* 1996; 6:107–127.
35. Blendon RJ, Szalay US, Knox RA. Should physicians aid their patients in dying? The public perspective. *JAMA* 1992; 267:2658–2662.
36. Graber MA, Levy BI, Weir RF, Oppliger RA. Patients' views about physician participation in assisted suicide and euthanasia. *J Gen Intern Med* 1996; 11:71–76.
37. Bachman JG, Alchser KH, Doukas DJ, Lichtenstein RL, Corning AD, Brody H. Attitudes of Michigan physicians and the public toward legalizing physician-assisted suicide and voluntary euthanasia. *N Engl J Med* 1996; 334:303–309.
38. Fried C. *Right and Wrong*. Cambridge, Mass.: Harvard University Press, 1978.
39. Nagel T. *The View from Nowhere*. Oxford, England: Oxford University Press, 1986.
40. Donagan A. *The Theory of Morality*. Chicago: University of Chicago, 1977.
41. Brody H. Causing, intending and assisting death. *J Clin Ethics* 1993; 4:112–117.
42. Meisel A. *The Right to Die*, 2nd ed. New York: Wiley, 1995.
43. Brock D. Death and Dying. In: Veatch RM, editor. *Medical Ethics*. Sudbury, Mass.: Jones and Bartlett, 1997, pp. 363–394.

12

Palliative Options of Last Resort:
A Comparison of Practices, Justifications,
and Safeguards

How should physicians respond to patients who are competent, terminally ill, and suffering in ways they find unacceptable in spite of excellent palliative care? Patients are clearly within their legal rights to ask for intensive management of pain and other symptoms, even if such treatment risks hastening death. They can also legally choose to stop all potentially life-sustaining therapy, even if their desire is for an earlier death. Unfortunately, some patients who have stopped all life-sustaining treatments continue to suffer intolerably in spite of state-of-the-art efforts at pain and symptom management, and do not die in what they consider a timely way.

This chapter begins with clinical illustrations and analysis of the widely accepted practices of intensive pain management and of stopping life supports. It then gives clinical examples and compares four additional potential interventions of last resort for competent terminally ill patients who are suffering intolerably (see Table 12–1). These latter four interventions should be considered only when intensive pain and symptom management is not working and all potential life-sustaining therapies have been stopped. Some clinicians and patients find the differences between these practices to be ethically and psychologically critical, whereas others perceive them as inconsequential. Voluntarily stopping eating and drinking and terminal sedation are legally accepted, and there is growing ethical consensus in the palliative care

TABLE 12–1. Potential Palliative Options of Last Resort

Legal Acceptability; Ethical Consensus; Standards of Practice

Intensive pain and symptom management

Not starting or stopping potentially life-sustaining therapy

Legal Acceptability; Growing Ethical Consensus

Voluntarily stopping eating and drinking (VSED)

Terminal sedation (TS)

Ethical Controversy; Legal Prohibition in Most States

Physician-assisted suicide (PAS)

Voluntary active euthanasia (VAE)

community about their appropriateness as a last-resort response.[1-3] In the United States, physician-assisted suicide has been legalized only in Oregon,[4] and voluntary active euthanasia is uniformly illegal. Despite their illegal status, both of these latter practices are used infrequently as a last resort to respond to otherwise intractable suffering, generally in secret without documentation or consultation.[5,6]

The recent Supreme Court decisions declaring that there is no constitutional right to physician-assisted suicide placed great emphasis on the importance of relieving pain and suffering near the end of life.[7,8] The Court acknowledged the legal acceptability of providing pain relief, even to the point of hastening death if necessary, and left open the possibility that states could legalize or prohibit physician-assisted suicide using other legal pathways. The Court, while choosing not to resolve the legal questions surrounding physician-assisted suicide, clearly wanted clinicians and policy makers to struggle on behalf of patients who have a compelling need and very few acceptable options.

Practices with Wide Legal and Ethical Acceptance

Standard Pain Management

A 68 year-old man with metastatic small cell lung cancer is experiencing excruciating bone pain, and is near death. He initially responded to a combination of radiation and chemotherapy, achieving a three-year remission. When his disease recurred four months previously, he elected a palliative approach. His pain from extensive bony metastases was initially well-controlled with high-dose, around-the-clock opioids, supplemented by radiation and nerve blocks. He prepared for death through talks with his family and clergy, and felt that he had no remaining "unfinished business." He now weighs 80 pounds and is bed bound, and his pain averages 8 on a 0–10 scale where 0 is "no pain" and 10 is "excruciating." He does not want to die, but is willing to accept the risks of sedation and an earlier death that might come from further increasing his doses of opioids. After a palliative care consultation, his physician increases the patient's total opioid doses by 25% per day until his pain is adequately controlled, or, if sedated, he appears comfortable.

On the third day the patient becomes very sleepy but arousable, and appears relatively free of pain. The physician shifts an equivalent amount of opioids from oral to transcutaneous routes, because the patient is unable to reliably swallow. The patient remains unresponsive, but appears comfortable. The dose of opioid is neither increased nor decreased until he dies two days later.

Standard pain management has wide social acceptance within medical, legal, and religious groups, and among the public.[9-15] For most of his illness, this patient's pain was well-controlled with high-dose opioids, and he was fully alert and functioning. When his pain accelerated toward the end, both patient and physician were willing to risk the possibility of an earlier death as an unintended side effect of intensive pain management, but it was not a hidden or explicit intent. The patient's suffering was severe enough to warrant taking the risk. Therefore, this action was consistent with the rule of double effect.[16] Had the patient's or the clinician's intent been to hasten death, justification using this rule would be more difficult.[17] Good pain management can usually be achieved without sedation and without shortening life; in fact, adequate control of pain is more likely to lengthen life than shorten it. However, sometimes pain is so severe or the patient is so frail, particularly right before death, that the risk of accelerating death is real. When this patient lapsed into a sleepy state, his dose of opioid was continued at the same level, and the side effect of sedation was accepted as proportionately necessary to control his pain.

Withdrawal of Life-Sustaining Treatment

A 56 year-old man had a malignant brain tumor that was diagnosed three years previously. He initially responded to a combination of surgery, radiation, chemotherapy, and corticosteroids. Although his cognitive abilities had diminished to a point where he could no longer work as an accountant, his altered brain unleashed new creativity in his hobby of painting. Later, when his tumor began to rapidly grow, he developed terrifying seizures and would feel paranoid, confused, and threatened. During his seizure-free times, he began talking in earnest about being ready to die. He was treated with anticonvulsants and antidepressants, with little relief. He tried unsuccesfully to end his life by jumping into Lake Ontario in winter, and was put on 24 hour "suicide watch."

His physician subsequently realized that his corticosteroid treatment was probably prolonging his life by preventing his brain from swelling, and that the patient could choose to discontinue it. After ethics and palliative care consultations, it was decided that providing this option was both morally acceptable and clinically appropriate. The patient was mentally capable of accepting or rejecting treatment, even that which was potentially life sustaining. Upon being given this choice, the patient immediately refused further corticosteroid treatment in the hope and expectation that he would die sooner rather than later. Within 12 hours, he went into a deep coma (probably from a combination of brain swelling and iatrogenic adrenal insufficiency). He had no pain or agitation, and died peacefully 24 hours later.

A patient's right to refuse life-sustaining treatment, or to stop it once started, has wide legal and ethical acceptance.[18–22] This right holds even if a patient wishes to die and could live indefinitely with the treatment, provided the patient is fully informed about the alternatives and has the mental capacity to understand the decision. Families can generally make these decisions on behalf of a patient who has lost mental capacity, provided there is a clear consensus that such actions reflect the patient's values, previously stated wishes, and best interests.[21] Because these decisions frequently result in the patient's death, clinicians should be forthright about evaluating such requests, carefully assessing the patient's mental capacity, the information about all palliative care alternatives, and the proportionate presence of suffering. This patient's wish to die was labeled "suicidal" until it was realized that he was within his rights to stop life supports, which allowed a more open-minded conversation between patient, family, physicians, and the health care team than had previously been possible.

Comparisons of Other Potential "Last-Resort" Practices

Voluntary Stopping of Eating and Drinking

An 83 year-old woman with degenerative joint disease, osteoporosis, and coronary artery disease experienced a major cerebrovascular accident that left her with a dense left-sided hemiparesis, but she retained cognition and speech. She stayed at home for the first year after her stroke with extensive support from her family, home health aide, and community health nurses.

Eventually, her personal health needs increased to the point that she was admitted to a skilled-nursing facility. Six months later, after lengthy discussions with her family, her doctor, and clergy, she stopped all of her medicines other than pain relievers, and adopted a purely palliative approach. Her care at the nursing facility was then supplemented by a hospice team. Her goal was to achieve a quicker end to what had become for her a seemingly interminable dying process. She initially felt elated by the decision, and began saying good-bye by telling life stories to her family in tape-recorded interviews. After three months of meaningful preparation, all the stories had been told, and she had again stabilized with what she viewed as a very poor quality of life.

She began talking in earnest about wanting to die. A lifelong Unitarian, she had no personal moral objection to voluntarily hastening death, but she refused to compromise anyone in her family or her physician given the current state of the law. She read a newspaper account of David Eddy's mother's decision to stop eating and drinking,[23] and immediately began exploring this option with her family and physician. Her family initially worried that it would be a long, painful process, but her doctor found some data about cancer patients dying this way that they found reassuring.[24] Several staff members were unable to accept her choice, and were reassigned to other patients.

As the process unfolded, her family visited every day in rotating shifts. The patient was initially very talkative, and had a special word for each of her children and grandchildren. On day six, she became sleepy and intermittently confused. The nursing staff kept her mouth moist and her skin well creamed. Her favorite music played constantly in the background. The staff was prepared to provide sedation if she became agitated or clearly uncomfortable, but this proved unnecessary. She was in a coma for the final three days of the 15-day process.

Voluntary stopping of eating and drinking (VSED) occurs when a patient who is otherwise physically capable of taking nourishment makes an active decision to discontinue all oral intake and is gradually "allowed to die" of dehydration or some intervening complication.[23,25,26] Depending on the patient's preexisting condition, this process usually takes one to three weeks—or longer if the patient continues to take some fluids. VSED has several advantages compared to other last-resort possibilities. Many patients lose their appetites and stop eating and drinking in the final stages of many illnesses. Ethically and legally, the right of competent, informed patients to refuse life-prolonging interventions, including artificial hydration and nutrition, is firmly established, and voluntary cessation of "natural" eating and drinking could be considered an extension of that right. There is, therefore, a growing consensus that the practice of VSED does not require a change in the law. Because it requires considerable discipline and time, the patient's persistent resolve to end his or her life is more assured. VSED also protects patient privacy and independence—so much so that it may require no participation by a physician.

The main disadvantages of VSED are that it may last for weeks and can initially increase suffering because the patient may experience thirst and hunger. Subtle coercion to proceed with the process may occur if patients are not regularly offered the opportunity to eat and drink, yet such offers may be viewed as undermining the patient's resolve. Some patients, family members, physicians, or nurses may find the notion of "dehydrating" or "starving" a patient to death to be morally repugnant. For patients whose immediate suffering is severe and unrelievable, the duration of the process would be unacceptable without accompanying sedation and analgesia. If physicians are not involved, palliation of symptoms may be inadequate, the decision to forgo eating and drinking may not be informed, and cases of treatable depression may be missed. Patients are likely to lose mental clarity toward the end of this process, which may undermine their sense of personal integrity or raise questions about whether the action remains voluntary.

Although several articles,[25,26] including a moving personal narrative,[23] have proposed VSED as an alternative to other forms of hastened death, there are no data that show how frequently such decisions are made or how acceptable they are to patients, families, physicians, or nurses.

Terminal Sedation

A 35 year-old man had had acquired immunodeficiency syndrome (AIDS) for more than 10 years. He had been near death several times over the last five years, and had been in an AIDS hospice when protease inhibitors became available. With the addition of protease inhibitors to his regimen, he recovered from recurrent infections and severe wasting to feel robust, gain weight, and return to his work as an interior designer for two years. However, over the next nine months, his disease again began progressing in spite of numerous medication adjustments. He started losing weight again, developed AIDS-related enteropathy, and began to lose his sight from long-standing CMV retinitis. This time, despite numerous changes in his antiretroviral regimen, there was no reprieve. He was again admitted to a residential hospice. He was very fearful of AIDS dementia, and was reassured by his physician that he could be sedated to unconsciousness if he became severely confused or agitated.

His initial time in the hospice program was comfortable and meaningful, as he had healing contact with family, friends, and clergy. As death approached, he developed high fevers, shaking chills, and increasing shortness of breath. These symptoms were treated with a morphine infusion and acetaminophen, but included no medical workup or antibiotic treatment. As his dose of morphine was increased in an effort to relieve his symptoms, he became delirious and agitated. The dose was decreased, and he awoke, but he was very uncomfortable. He requested that his doctor help him escape from his agony. The doctor offered to sedate him to unconsciousness, then withhold further treatments, including intravenous fluids. The patient was reassured that the dose would be increased until he appeared to be resting comfortably, and that it would not be cut back until he died. A consensus that this was the best of the available options was reached among the health care team, the patient, and the family. It would allow the patient to achieve a wished-for death without violating the law or forcing him to suffer unnecessarily. He was put on a midazolam infusion, which was gradually increased until he achieved a sedated state, and then maintained at that level. He died within 24 hours.

Terminal sedation (TS) occurs when a suffering patient is sedated to unconsciousness, usually through the ongoing administration of barbiturates or benzodiazepines. The patient then dies of dehydration, starvation, or some other intervening complication, as all life-sustaining interventions are withheld.[3,27–29] Although death is inevitable, it usually does not take place for days or even weeks, depending on the clinical circumstances. Because patients are deeply sedated during this terminal period, they are believed to be free of suffering. It can be argued that death with TS is "foreseen" but not "intended" and that the sedation itself is not causing death.[27–29] The sedation is intended to relieve suffering, a long-standing and uncontroversial aim of medicine, and the subsequent withholding of life-sustaining therapy has wide legal and ethical acceptance. Thus, performing TS probably requires no change in the law, and the recent Supreme Court decisions give strong support to TS, saying that pain in terminally ill patients should be treated, even to the point of rendering the patient unconscious or hastening death.[7,8] Terminal sedation is already openly practiced by some palliative care and hospice groups in cases of unrelieved suffering, with a reported frequency of 0%–44% of cases.[3,14,27–33]

Terminal sedation has other practical advantages. It can be carried out in patients with severe physical limitations. The time delay between initiation of TS and death permits second-guessing and reassessment by the health care team and the family. Because the health care team must administer medications and monitor effects, physicians can ensure that the patient's decision is informed and voluntary before beginning TS. In addition, many proponents believe that it is appropriate to use TS for patients who lack decision-making capacity and whose suffering is extreme and otherwise unrelievable, with the consent of the patient's designated surrogate or family.

Nonetheless, TS remains controversial[34-36] and has many of the same risks associated with voluntary active euthanasia (VAE) and physician-assisted suicide (PAS). As with VAE, the final actors are the clinicians, not the patient. Terminal sedation could therefore be carried out without explicit discussions with alert patients who appear to be suffering intolerably. It may even be against their wishes. Some competent, terminally ill patients reject TS. They believe that their dignity would be violated if they had to be unconscious for a prolonged time before they die, or that their families would suffer unnecessarily while waiting for them to die. Patients who wish to die in their own homes may not be able to arrange for TS, because it usually requires admission to a health care facility. There is also some controversy in the anesthesia literature about whether heavily sedated persons are actually free of suffering or simply are unable to report or remember it.[37-39] There are also some clinical situations where TS is insufficient to relieve a patient's symptoms, and therefore other options may be needed (e.g., uncontrollable bleeding from an eroding lesion or a refractory coagulation disorder, an inability to swallow secretions from widespread oropharyngeal cancer, or refractory diarrhea from acquired immunodeficiency syndrome). Although such patients are probably not conscious of their condition once sedated, their death is unlikely to be dignified or remembered as peaceful by their families. Finally, and perhaps most critically, there may be confusion about the physician's ethical responsibility in contributing to a patient's death.[34,35]

Physician-Assisted Suicide*

A 59 year-old man had oropharyngeal cancer that was diagnosed two years previously. His tumor was too large to be resected, so he was treated with chemotherapy and radiation. He was relatively asymptomatic for one year during which he worked his usual job. Then his tumor recurred inside his mouth and in his neck, making it hard for him to swallow his secretions. His initial goal was to live as long as his symptoms could be adequately

---

* The term "physician-assisted suicide" is used here to describe this practice because of its widespread use in the medical literature. However, the concept of suicide does not accurately reflect the meaning of this action, nor does it necessarily differentiate it from other last-resort practices. Technically, five of the six cases presented here might be considered suicide in the sense that death was being sought by the patient as the only means to escape intolerable suffering. However, "suicide" also connotes an act of self-destructiveness by a person with mental illness, whereas in each of these cases, seeking death was viewed by the patients as a form of self-preservation. We must make sure that politicized public discussion about the legalization of this practice does not lead to distortion of the issues, and ultimately to uninformed decision making.

managed, then to die as quickly and painlessly as possible. He was particularly afraid of suffocation, which he had seen in a coworker who died of emphysema. His pain was well-controlled with around-the-clock administration of sustained-release morphine. He was admitted to a home hospice program.

His time in hospice was very meaningful, with regular visits from members of his church congregation, friends, and hospice workers, in addition to his family. Unfortunately, his tumor eventually began to bleed profusely both inside his mouth and outside his neck. He was terrified of suffocating and bleeding to death. He asked for enough barbiturates to "put me out of my misery." He considered stopping eating and drinking, but felt the wait for dehydration to death would be too long given his current acutely deteriorating condition. He was offered terminal sedation so that he could escape his suffering, but he remained fearful of bleeding out and suffocating, and not being able to tell his caregivers about his subjective state. He was also worried about the impact on his family of their watching him bleed to death. His family understood and accepted his decision, and was willing to support him in the process if his physician was willing to provide a prescription for barbiturates. After discussing the situation with his practice partners, the physician reluctantly but knowingly provided him with a lethal amount of barbiturates in a prescription ostensibly intended for insomnia. That evening, the patient took the entire amount with his family present, went into a deep sleep, and died quietly. Because the practice was illegal in the patient's home state, there was no documentation of the patient's final hours.

Physician-assisted suicide (PAS) occurs when a physician provides the means, usually a prescription for a large dose of barbiturates, by which a patient can end his or her life.[14,15,40] Although the physician is morally responsible for this assistance, the patient carries out the final act. Physician-assisted suicide has several advantages. For some patients, access to a lethal dose of medication may give them the freedom and reassurance to continue living, knowing they can escape if and when they choose.[41,42] Because patients have to ingest the drug by their own hand, the action is likely to be voluntary. Physicians report being more comfortable with PAS than VAE,[43-45] presumably because their participation is indirect.

Opponents of PAS believe that it violates traditional moral and professional prohibitions against intentionally contributing to a patient's death. Physician-assisted suicide also has several practical disadvantages. Self-administration does not guarantee competence or voluntariness. The patient may have impaired judgment at the time of the request, or the act may be influenced by external pressures. Physician-assisted suicide is also limited to patients who are physically capable of taking medication themselves. It is not always effective,[46-48] so families may be faced with a patient who is vomiting, aspirating, or cognitively impaired, but not dying. Patients brought to an emergency department after an ineffective attempt are likely to receive unwanted life-prolonging treatment. Requiring the presence of a physician when a patient ingests the medication could have the unintended consequence of being coercive as to the timing of the act, yet the absence of a physician may force families to respond to medical complications alone.

Physician-assisted suicide is illegal in most states; however, no physician has ever been successfully prosecuted for this crime.[15] In Chapter 13, the limited data about the practice in the United States will be reviewed, as will two years of data from Oregon, where PAS has recently been legalized.

Voluntary Active Euthanasia

A 79 year-old Dutch woman had end-stage congestive heart failure. She had lived alone in a small apartment in Utrecht since her husband died 10 years before. Her son and daughter lived nearby, visiting regularly and helping with her care. She was able to fix her own meals, and dress and toilet herself, but she was too weak and easily fatigued to do much else. She was adamant about not going to a nursing home. "I would rather die in my own bed," she would say. On a daily basis, she required 10 different medications, a total of 48 pills per day. Her family physician (*huisart*) lived in the neighborhood, and each week would visit her at home for support and medication adjustment. They had several long talks about her view of her declining quality of life and her fears about suffocation, and she queried him about his views on euthanasia. The physician said that he had an open mind about euthanasia if all else failed, but he hoped that they would be able to manage her medical problems sufficiently without it.

She had had several heart attacks over the last eight years. In the previous six months, she had been admitted to the hospital five times with severe pulmonary edema. In her next-to-last hospitalization, she was put on a mechanical ventilator for over a week, and she found the experience to be terrifying. She and her physician agreed to not provide mechanical ventilation again, but this left the challenge of how to respond when she next went into heart failure. They agreed to provide morphine to help alleviate her shortness of breath, and diuretics to try to mobilize the fluid, but she remained fearful about just how this would work since her symptoms often came on suddenly and severely.

One week later she again went into acute heart failure, and was brought to the hospital and given morphine and diuretics. After several hours she mobilized the fluid, and she was eventually sent home with some additional medication. Once home, she became adamant that her current situation was intolerable. Her view was that her quality of life was poor, and she was dreading the next episode of heart failure, which might or might not end her life. She talked with her children about requesting euthanasia. They were initially against it, but after many long talks they reluctantly agreed. The patient and her family then asked that the family physician visit to discuss these issues. They explored all alternatives, including stopping all her medications and then sedating her as the shortness of breath started, or more aggressive sedation when the next episode occurred. The patient saw no sense in waiting to again go into heart failure with its associated severe symptoms, or precipitating heart failure by stopping her medication. "Why not just let me die without enduring more suffering?"

The Dutch doctor asked a colleague to visit the patient at home to make sure that she was clear about her wishes, that all alternatives had been explored, and that all criteria had been met. The patient and family then selected a date one week later. During the last week, the patient settled her remaining financial affairs and said good-bye to friends and family. At the agreed-upon time, her children, several close friends, and her pastor were present. Her family physician came to her home and made sure she was clear about her wishes. Then he started an intravenous line and administered a sedating dose of barbiturates. Once she was deeply sleeping, he administered a muscle-paralyzing agent that stopped her breathing. She died several minutes later. The family, friends, and family physician stayed together for the next hour and reminisced about the patient's life.

Voluntary active euthanasia (VAE) occurs when a physician administers a lethal injection at a patient's request.[9,14] As practiced in the Netherlands, the patient is sedated to unconsciousness and is then given a lethal injection of a muscle-paralyzing agent like curare. For patients who are prepared to die because their suffering is intolerable, VAE has the advantage of being quick and effective. Patients need not have manual dexterity, the ability to swallow, or an intact gastrointestinal system. It also requires active and direct physician participation. This is beneficial in that physicians can check the patient's competence and voluntariness at the time of the act, support the family, and respond to complications. The directness of the act makes the physician's moral responsibility clear.

On the other hand, VAE explicitly and directly conflicts with traditional medical prohibitions against intentionally causing death.[49] Furthermore, it can be conducted without explicit patient consent.[50,51] For example, VAE could be used on patients who appear to be suffering severely or posing extreme burdens to their physician, family, or society, but who have lost the mental capacity to make informed decisions.

The Netherlands is the only country where both VAE and PAS are openly practiced, regulated, and studied. Both practices remain technically illegal in the Netherlands, but they are not prosecuted provided that participating physicians adhere to the agreed-upon guidelines.[52] Chapter 13 compares the ethical, legal, and clinical climates surrounding end-of-life practices in the Netherlands and the United States, and explains how the Dutch tolerate the ambiguous legal status of these two practices. It will also provide an overview of the findings of the two Remmelink studies, in which all end-of-life practices in the Netherlands were systematically reviewed.[53,54]

United States laws prohibiting VAE are stricter than those governing PAS, and a physician is more likely to be prosecuted for participating in this practice. Physicians also appear to be more reluctant to participate in VAE even if it were legal.[43,44] Voluntary active euthanasia was recently legalized in a province of Australia, but this legalization was subsequently reversed by the legislature.[55]

Additional Discussion About the Cases

Although the case studies presented here portray clear distinctions among six last-resort interventions (see Table 12–1), in practice both the clinical indications and the practices may blur. Categorization may depend on specific circumstances, and may be subject to interpretation. For example, the distinction between terminal sedation and voluntary active euthanasia is based in part on whether the dose of a sedative is maintained or increased once sedation is achieved, and whether a lethal injection is given. Differences are also based on the physician's intent to hasten death, which is subjective and never absolutely knowable.[17,56] Reasonable observers might differ in their categorization of terminal sedation with respect to physician intent, especially if a patient selects this option to escape suffering and hasten inevitable death.[2,35] Similarly, what begins as voluntarily stopping eating and drinking in an alert, capable patient may become withholding life supports from an incompetent patient as obtundation occurs. If a patient subsequently becomes delirious in this terminal phase, VSED might have to be followed by terminal sedation.[2] Experienced clinicians could easily think of other examples where the health care team and the family might be hard-pressed to find a suitable approach.

In the setting of severe, otherwise unrelievable suffering that is unacceptable to the dying patient, each of these interventions alone or in combination may have a small place. Only in the first case, that illustrating standard pain management, was death clearly unintended by both patient and physician—the risk of death was understood given the grave condition of the patient, but it was not the goal of either party. The second patient hoped for death as a means of escaping suffering and stopped corticosteroid therapy, but this outcome was not a certainty. With the other four interventions, death was the inevitable outcome and was clearly sought by the patients. Although the physician's purpose in participating in these alternatives is to respond to human suffering, the decision-making process should include acknowledgment that the patient's death is inevitable. In any of these interventions, a participating physician must ensure the adequacy of palliative care, a full exploration of alternatives, a complete evaluation of the patient's mental capacity, and the proportionate presence of suffering.

Standard pain management and the stopping of life-sustaining therapy are standards of care, and all clinicians should be willing to provide them. Even though terminal sedation and voluntarily stopping eating and drinking are legal, they should be considered only when no acceptable palliative care alternatives are available, and when both patient and physician consider them to be morally acceptable. Physician-assisted suicide remains illegal in most states, although it is not vigorously sought out or prosecuted provided it remains outside of public view. PAS should be exceedingly rare, performed only on request from a terminally ill patient whose suffering is intolerable, and when other alternatives are inadequate or incompatible with the patient's fundamental values. Voluntary active euthanasia is a legally tolerated option in the Netherlands, but in the United States the practice is more likely to be vigorously and successfully prosecuted than physician-assisted suicide.°

None of these solutions is perfect. The challenge for the patient, family, and health care team is to find the "least worst" solution given the values of the participants and the patient's clinical situation, and keeping in mind the relevant local laws.[57] Physicians who unilaterally choose not to select one of these options are obligated to search for acceptable alternatives with the patient. Ethics and palliative care consults may be helpful. If a mutually acceptable approach cannot be found, the patient and family should be given the option of transferring care to another physician.

Ethical Justifications and Comparisons

Many normative ethical analyses use the doctrine of double effect and the distinction between active and passive assistance to evaluate acts that may

_____

° Jack Kevorkian flouted the law prohibiting physician-assisted suicide, and was unable to be successfully prosecuted. However, when he performed voluntary active euthanasia, he was relatively quickly convicted and sent to jail.

TABLE   12–2. Potential   Ethical   Justifications   for Last-Resort Practices

---

- Rule of double effect
- Active/passive distinction
- Voluntariness
- Proportionality
- Conflict of duties

---

hasten death and are currently permissible (forgoing life-sustaining treatment and high-dose pain medications) and those that are impermissible (PAS and VAE).[9,10,14,58,59] Both TS and VSED are considered to be ethically preferable alternatives to PAS and VAE on the basis of similar arguments.[25–27,32] In this section, these arguments are critically examined. Issues of voluntariness, proportionality, and conflict of duties are presented as more central and less problematic to the ethical evaluation of these options than the doctrine of double effect or the active/passive distinction. The discussion is restricted to the potential ethical permissibility of these actions, not their public policy implications. Table 12–2 summarizes the potential ethical justifications considered in this discussion.

Rule of Double Effect

As discussed in Chapter 11, when evaluating an action, the rule of double effect distinguishes among effects that a person intends (both the end sought and the means taken to the end) and consequences that are foreseen but un-intended.[34,35,60,61] As long as a physician's intentions are good, it is permissible to perform actions with foreseeable consequences that it would be wrong to intend. In this view, intentionally causing death is morally impermissible, even if it is desired by a competent patient whose suffering cannot be relieved otherwise. However, if death comes unintentionally as a consequence of an otherwise well-intentioned intervention, even if it can easily be foreseen, the physician's action can be morally acceptable. The unintended but foreseen bad effect must also be proportional to the intended good effect. Elements of the rule of double effect are summarized in Table 11–1 in the preceding chapter.

The rule of double effect has been important in justifying the use of pain medications to relieve suffering near the end of life.[9,10,14,58,59] When high-dose opioids are used to treat pain, neither the patient nor the physician intends to accelerate death. The risk of unintentionally hastening death in order to relieve pain is accepted. The rule of double effect has also been used to distinguish TS from PAS and VAE.[3,27,29,32] Relief of suffering is intended in all three options, but death is argued to be intended with PAS and VAE but merely foreseen with

TS. However, it seems implausible to claim that death is unintended when a patient who wants to die is sedated to the point of coma, and intravenous fluids and artificial nutrition are withheld, making death certain.[34,35,56] Although the overarching intention of the sedation is to relieve the patient's suffering, the additional step of withholding fluids and nutrition is not needed to relieve pain but is typically performed to hasten the patient's wished-for death. In contrast, when patients are sedated to treat conditions like status epilepticus, therapies such as fluids and mechanical ventilation are continued with the goal of prolonging life.

The rule of double effect puts particular moral emphasis on the intention of the physician. Having a physician intentionally end a patient's life is always morally impermissible, no matter how desperate the patient's clinical situation or how directly the patient is requesting assistance, yet ending life foreseeably but unintentionally can be permissible when it produces a proportionate good. An alternative view is to place the foremost emphasis on the patient's will and clinical situation. It would always be morally wrong to end the life of a person who wants to live, whether doing so intentionally or foreseeably. What can make TS morally permissible according to this point of view is that the patient gives informed consent to it, not that the physician only foresees but does not intend the patient's inevitable death.

The issue of intention is complicated because determining what is intended by the patient or physician is often difficult to verify, and because practices that are universally accepted may involve the intent to hasten death in some cases.[34,62] Death is not always intended or sought when competent patients forgo life support; sometimes patients simply do not want to continue a particular treatment but hope they can live without it. However, some patients find their circumstances intolerable even with the best of care, and refuse further life support with the intent of bringing about their death. There is broad agreement that physicians must respect such refusals, even when the patient's intention is to die.[9,10,14,15,58,59,62] However, such practices are highly problematic when analyzed according to the doctrine of double effect.

The Active/Passive Distinction

According to many normative ethical analyses, active measures that hasten death are unacceptable, whereas passive or indirect measures that achieve the same ends may be permitted.[9,10,14,58,59,63] How this active/passive distinction applies to these last-resort practices remains controversial.[34,35] Voluntary active euthanasia provides active assistance in dying—that is, a physician's actions directly cause a patient's death. Stopping life-sustaining therapies is typically considered passive assistance in dying, as the patient is said to die of the disease no matter how proximate the physician's action is to the patient's death. However, physicians sometimes experience stopping life-sustaining interventions as very active.[64] For example, there is nothing psychologically or physically passive about taking off a mechanical ventilator someone who is incapable of breathing on his or her own. Voluntarily stopping eating and drinking is argued to be a variant of stopping life-sustaining therapy, and the patient is said to die of the disease.[25,26] The notion that VSED passively "lets nature take its course" is unpersuasive, because patients with no underlying disease would also die if they stopped eating and drinking. Death is more a result of the patient's will and resolve than an inevitable consequence of his disease. Furthermore, even if the physician's role in hastening death is generally passive or indirect, most would argue that it is desirable to have physicians involved to actively palliate symptoms and make sure that the patient is fully informed.

Both PAS and TS are difficult to evaluate according to the active/passive distinction. Physician-assisted suicide is active in that the physician provides the means whereby the patient may end his or her life and thereby contributes to an immediate cause of death different from the patient's disease. However, the physician's role in PAS is passive or indirect, because the patient administers the lethal medication. This psychological and temporal distance between providing a prescription and the act itself may make PAS seem indirect, more ambiguous, and thereby more acceptable to physicians than VAE.[43–45]

Terminal sedation is passive, because the administration of sedation does not directly cause a patient's death and because withholding artificial feedings and fluids is considered passively allowing the patient to die.[3,27,32] However, some physicians and nurses may consider it very active to sedate to unconsciousness someone who is seeking death and then to withhold life-prolonging interventions. Furthermore, the notion that TS is merely "letting nature take its course" is problematic. Often a patient dies of dehydration from the withholding of fluids, not from the underlying disease.

The application and the moral significance of both the active/passive distinction and the doctrine of double effect are notoriously controversial and should not serve as the primary basis for determining the ethical propriety of these practices.

Voluntariness

It seems clear that the patient's wishes and consent are more ethically important than whether the method is categorized as active or passive or whether death is intended or unintended by the physician.[65–67] With competent patients, none of these acts would be morally permissible without the patient's voluntary and informed consent. Any of these actions would violate a competent patient's autonomy and would be both immoral and illegal if the patient did not understand that death was the inevitable consequence of the action or if the decision was coerced or contrary to the patient's wishes. The ethical principle of autonomy focuses on patients' rights to make important decisions about their lives, including what happens to their bodies, and may support genuinely autonomous forms of these acts.[40,63]

However, because most of these acts require cooperation from physicians and, in the case of TS, the health care team, the autonomy of participating medical professionals also warrants consideration. Because TS, VSED, PAS, and VAE are not part of usual medical practice and all result in a hastened death, clinicians should have the right to determine the nature and extent of their own participation. All physicians should respect patients' decisions to forgo life-sustaining treatment, including artificial hydration and nutrition, and provide standard palliative care, including skillful pain and symptom management. If society permits some or all of these practices (currently TS and VSED are openly tolerated), physicians who choose not to participate because of personal moral considerations should at a minimum discuss all available alternatives in the interest of informed patient consent and respect for patient autonomy. Physicians are free to express their own objections to these practices as part of the informing process, to propose alternative approaches, and to transfer care to another physician if the patient continues to request actions to hasten death that they find unacceptable.

Proportionality

The ethical principles of beneficence and nonmaleficence obligate the physician to act in a patient's best interests and to avoid causing net harm.[63] The concept of proportionality requires that the risk of causing harm bear a direct relationship to the danger and immediacy of a patient's clinical situation and the expected benefit of the interventions.[63,68] The greater the patient's suffering, the greater risk a physician can take in potentially contributing to the patient's death, as long as the patient understands and accepts that risk. For a patient with lung cancer who is anxious and short of breath, the risk in prescribing small doses of morphine or anxiolytics is warranted. At a later time, if a patient is near death and gasping for air, more aggressive sedation is indicated, even in doses that may well cause respiratory depression. Although proportionality is an important element of the rule of double effect, it can be applied independent of this rule. Sometimes a patient's suffering cannot be relieved despite optimal palliative care, and continuing to live causes torment that can end only with death.[69] Such extreme circumstances sometimes warrant extraordinary medical actions, and the means of hastening death under consideration in this chapter may satisfy the requirement of proportionality. The requirement of proportionality, which all health care interventions should meet, does not support any principled ethical distinction between these options.

Conflict of Duties

Unrelievable, intolerable suffering by patients at the end of life may create for physicians a conflict between their ethical and professional duty to relieve suffering and their ethical and professional duty not to use at least some means to deliberately hasten death.[52,69] Physicians who believe they should respond to such suffering by acceding to the patient's request for a hastened death may find themselves caught between their duty to the patient as a caregiver and their duty to obey the law as a citizen.[68] Solutions often can be found in the intensive application of palliative care, or in the currently legitimized options of forgoing life supports, VSED, or TS. In some cases, these options may not be adequate or acceptable. Clearly, the physician has a moral obligation not to abandon patients with unrelieved suffering;[70] hence, those physicians who cannot provide some or all of these options because of moral or legal reservations should be required to search assiduously with the patient for mutually acceptable solutions.

Safeguards

Safeguards to protect vulnerable patients from the risk of error, abuse, or coercion must be in place for each last-resort practice that is accepted or tolerated. This is particularly important in the United States, where health care is undergoing a radical reform based more on market forces than on a commitment to quality of care,[63,64] and 43 million persons are uninsured. Risks that have been cited in the debates about PAS and VAE[49-51] also exist for TS and VSED, as well as for forgoing life-sustaining therapy. Any of these practices can be carried out without ensuring that optimal palliative care has been provided. Physicians who believe that death is completely unintended with any of these practices may fail to acknowledge the inevitable consequences of their action or their responsibility.

Safeguards should be flexible enough to be responsive to individual patient dilemmas and rigorous enough to protect vulnerable persons. Categories of safeguards are summarized in Table 12–3, and include the following:

TABLE 12–3. Categories of Safeguards for Last Resort Practices: Patients with and without Decision-Making Capacity

---

Patients with Decision-Making Capacity

1. Effective palliative care
2. Intolerable suffering: proportionately severe to warrant life-ending intervention
3. Fully informed consent about condition, prognosis, and options
4. Diagnostic and prognostic clarity
5. Independent second opinion(s)
6. Clear documentation and review

Patients without Decision-Making Capacity°

1. Effective palliative care
2. Intolerable suffering: proportionately severe to warrant life-ending intervention
3. Patient clearly incapable of informed consent; person designated to represent the patient according to the following hierarchy:
   • A formally designated heath care proxy, or statements in a living will
   • Close family members using the principle of "substituted judgment"
   • Close family members representing the patient's "best interests"
   • A court-appointed guardian only if the options above fail to represent the patient
4. Diagnostic and prognostic clarity
5. Independent second opinion(s)
6. Clear documentation and review

° Voluntary stopping of eating and drinking, physician-assisted suicide, and voluntary active euthanasia are categorically excluded for patients without decision-making capacity, as voluntary consent is an absolute requirement for these three last-resort options.

1. *Effective palliative care*: Excellent palliative care must be available to every dying patient as a basic standard of care.
2. *Intolerable suffering*: A patient's suffering must be severe enough to warrant a potentially life-ending intervention, and must not be responsive to more standard palliative treatments.
3. *Informed consent*: A patient must be fully informed about his or her condition, prognosis, and treatment alternatives, including more conventional palliative alternatives. A patient's request for a hastened death must be clear and rational, free of undue influence, and enduring.
4. *Diagnostic and prognostic clarity*: A patient must have a clearly diagnosed disease with known lethality. The prognosis must be clearly understood by the patient and the physician, and include the degree of uncertainty about outcomes (i.e., how long the patient might live).
5. *Independent second opinion(s)*: A consultant with expertise in palliative care should review each case. Specialists should also review any questions

about the patient's diagnosis or prognosis. A psychiatrist should be consulted if there is uncertainty about treatable depression or about the patient's mental capacity.

6. *Documentation and review*: The clinical reasoning and support for each agreed-upon criterion should be carefully documented. Well-defined processes for documentation, reporting, and review should be in place to ensure accountability.

For patients who have lost the ability to make decisions for themselves, these last-resort decisions are even more daunting. Physicians have an obligation to respond to extremes of suffering in all of their dying patients, including those who cannot offer informed consent themselves. The three last-resort practices for which the voluntary consent of a competent patient is an absolute requirement—voluntary stopping eating and drinking, physician-assisted suicide, and voluntary active euthanasia—are clearly not possible for these patients. Standard pain management and similar treatment of symptoms such as shortness of breath are clearly required for incapacitated patients as part of basic palliative care.[9] A physician also has the right to refuse life-sustaining treatment on behalf of a patient if stopping or not starting treatment is consistent with what is known about the patient's values and best interests.[21] There is a growing consensus among practitioners of palliative care and in debates on medical ethics that terminal sedation should be the response of last resort for patients with even the most advanced terminal symptoms, including patients with agitated terminal delirium.[2,3]

The safeguards for potentially life-ending decisions outlined above must be adapted for patients who lack the ability to make decisions for themselves, as follows:

1. The patient must be clearly incapable of making decisions for him- or herself, and therefore not able to offer informed consent. The patient should be evaluated by a mental health professional if there is uncertainty about his or her capacity to engage in decision making. If there is a reasonable chance that the patient can regain capacity to fully participate in decision making in the near future, then such last-resort interventions should be postponed if there is uncertainty about the patient's wishes.

2. Decision makers should be designated who can best represent the patient's interests and values. There is general agreement about the ethicality of the following hierarchical approach:[59,71]
   • If a patient has formally designated a health care proxy, this person should be empowered to make decisions on the patient's behalf using what is known about the patient's values and wishes.[58,59] If a living will exists, this should also guide decision making as it applies to the patient's current clinical situation.

- If there is no designated proxy or living will (as is the case the vast majority of the time), close family members should represent the patient as best they can, using the ethical principle of "substituted judgment" (i.e., to make decisions as they believe the patient would, using what is known about the patient's values and beliefs.)[58,59] It is acknowledged that substituted judgment is an inexact science,[72,73] but there is also general agreement that close family members are in the best position to represent the patient[74,75] and to communicate with providers of medical care.
- If nothing is known about the patient's values and wishes under the circumstances, then family members should try to represent the patient's "best interests." In Chapter 8, a process for achieving consensus on these matters is described.[76]
- Only when there is no family or loved ones available to represent the patient (or if those present cannot represent the patient's interests because of preexisting problems) should a court-appointed guardian be solicited.

The typical safeguards proposed for regulating VAE and PAS[77–80] attempt to put these principles into practice; they are intended to allow physicians to respond to unrelieved suffering while ensuring that adequate palliative measures have been attempted and that patient decisions are autonomous. Tables 13–1 and 13–2 in Chapter 13 summarize how these categories have been codified in Oregon and the Netherlands, where last-resort practices are regulated. Such safeguards must balance a respect for patient privacy with the need to adequately oversee these interventions.

Similar safeguards should be considered for TS and VSED, even if these practices are already sanctioned by the law. Table 12–4 presents proposed guidelines for TS and VSED based on published literature that is supported by a consensus panel assembled by the American College of Physicians–American Society of Internal Medicine.[2]

The restriction of any of these methods to the terminally ill involves a trade-off. Some patients who suffer greatly from incurable, but not terminal, illnesses and who are unresponsive to palliative measures will be denied access to a hastened death and forced to continue suffering against their will. Other patients whose request for a hastened death is denied will avoid a premature death because their suffering can subsequently be relieved with more intensive palliative care. Some methods (e.g., PAS, VAE, TS) might be restricted to the terminally ill because of current inequities of access, concerns about errors and abuse, and lack of experience with the process. VSED might be allowed for those who are incurably ill, but not facing imminent death, if they meet all other criteria. VSED might be considered under such circumstances because of its inherent waiting period and the time it allows for reconsideration, the great

TABLE 12–4. Potential Guidelines for Terminal Sedation and Voluntary Stopping of Eating and Drinking[a]

GUIDELINE DOMAIN	TERMINAL SEDATION	VOLUNTARY STOPPING OF EATING AND DRINKING
Palliative Care	Must be available, in place, and unable to relieve current suffering adequately	Must be available, in place, and unable to relieve current suffering adequately
Usual Patient Characteristics	1) Severe, immediate, otherwise unrelievable symptoms: (e.g. pain, shortness of breath, nausea, vomiting, seizures, delirium) 2) Can be used to prevent severe suffering: (e.g. to prevent suffocation sensation when discontinuing mechanical ventilation)	Persistent, unrelenting, otherwise unrelievable symptoms unacceptable to the patient: (e.g. extreme fatigue, weakness, debility)
Terminal Prognosis	Usually days to weeks	Usually weeks to months
Patient Informed Consent	Patient competent, fully informed; noncompetent with severe, otherwise irreversible suffering (use advance directive, and/or consensus about patient wishes and best interests)	Patient competent, fully informed
Family Participation in Decision	Strongly encourage input from and consensus of immediate family members	Strongly encourage input from and consensus of immediate family members
Incompetent Patient	Available for indications of severe, persistent suffering with the informed consent of the patient's designated proxy, family members. If no surrogate available, consensus from team members and consultants that no other acceptable palliative responses are available	Food and drink (oral food and fluids) must not be withheld from incompetent persons willing and able to eat
Second Opinion(s)	Expert in palliative care Mental health expert (if uncertainty about mental capacity)	Expert in palliative care Mental health expert Specialist in the patient's underlying disease (strongly advised)
Medical Staff Participation in Decision	Input from staff involved in immediate patient care activities encouraged; physician and staff consent for their own participation required	Input from staff involved in immediate patient care activities encouraged; physician and staff consent for their own participation required

[a]This table was originally presented in Quill TE, Byock IR. Responding to intractable terminal suffering: the role of terminal sedation and voluntary refusal of food and fluids. *Ann Int Med* 2000; 132:408–414. Reprinted with permission.

resolve it requires, and the fact that it does not require a physician's direct involvement. If any methods are extended to severely ill patients who are not facing imminent death, safeguards should be more stringent and include substantial waiting periods and mandatory assessment by psychiatrists and specialists. The risk of error in offering any of these last-resort options to this group of patients is increased, yet the consequences of not listening and responding to compelling cases are also substantial.

The clinical, ethical, and policy differences and similarities among these practices need to be debated openly, both publicly and within the medical profession. Some may worry that a discussion of the similarities between VSED and TS, on the one hand, and PAS and VAE, on the other, may undermine the desired goal of optimal relief of suffering at the end of life by making VSED and TS less available than they currently are.[40,41] Others may worry that a critical analysis of the principle of double effect or the active/passive distinction as applied to VSED and TS may undermine efforts to improve pain relief or to ensure that the patient's or surrogate's decisions to forgo unwanted life-sustaining therapy are respected.[81] However, hidden ambiguous practices, inconsistent justifications, and a failure to acknowledge the risks of accepted practices may also undermine the quality of terminal care and put patients at unnecessary risk.

Any of these last-resort options should be considered only in the context of good palliative care, and as small but important facets of comprehensive care for all dying patients.[9,10,14,15] Currently, TS and VSED are legal and are widely accepted by hospice and palliative care physicians. However, they may not be readily available, because some physicians may continue to have moral objections and legal fears about these options. Physician-assisted suicide is illegal in almost every state but Oregon. It may be difficult, if not impossible, to successfully prosecute if it is carried out at the request of an informed, terminally ill, suffering patient. Voluntary active euthanasia is illegal everywhere and is likely to be aggressively prosecuted if uncovered.

Explicit public policies about which of these practices are permissible and under what circumstances could have important benefits. Those who fear a difficult death would face the end of life knowing that their physicians can respond openly if their worst fears materialize. For most, reassurance will be all that is needed, because good palliative care is generally effective. Explicit guidelines for the practices that are deemed permissible can also encourage clinicians to explore why a patient requests hastening of death, to search for palliative care alternatives, and to respond to those whose suffering is greatest.[68]

Concluding Thoughts

Many patients have excellent pain control and quality of life for the majority of their clinical course, only to have symptoms accelerate and threats to their personhood intensify just prior to death. The sense of purpose, caring, and human connection achieved by patients and their loved ones during this period may be threatened and undermined if such severe symptoms and suffering in late stages are not adequately addressed. In-depth narratives describing patients' and families' experiences throughout the entire dying process, including the post-death bereavement period, may help us better understand the complex realities faced by dying patients and their families.[82] When patients die in the midst of unrelieved terminal struggle and distress, their families frequently wonder why this has happened to them. Questions are raised about the commitment and skill of the medical caregivers, as well as the compassion of a higher power that would allow this to occur. Sometimes images of an intractable, terrifying dilemma that arose just before death can haunt memories of more meaningful times, complicating grieving and intensifying fears of family members about their own deaths.

Instead of doing their utmost to respond, health care providers often become overly cautions in the face of severe terminal suffering. This stems in part from their personal ambivalence about the nearness of death,[83] but also from confusion about their responsibilities in balancing the relief of suffering and the prolongation of life as death approaches.[49,84] These are the moments when in-depth knowledge of aggressive pain management,[9,85] the doctrine of double effect,[16,17] the right to stop life-sustaining therapy,[18–21] and other last-resort options discussed in this chapter become important. Not joining with the patient and family at this point in an intensive search to find a mutually satisfactory solution may be a form of abandonment. The challenge is to respond in a way that is proportionate to the patient's suffering and responsive to the particulars of the patient's clinical condition and personal values. Clinicians must look within their own moral framework and experience as they try to deal compassionately and creatively with these patients, without violating their own beliefs and values. Their knowledge and expertise in palliative care must be supplemented with a working knowledge of these last-resort options, including some decision about how they plan to approach the most difficult cases.[86] Getting expert help from clinicians who are experienced in palliative care and ethics can be useful when it appears that there are no acceptable approaches.

- *Note*: Some of the material in this chapter comes from two previously published manuscripts. The first, coauthored by Bernie Lo and Dan Brock and titled "Palliative options of last resort: A comparison of voluntarily stopping eating and drinking, terminal sedation, physician-assisted suicide, and voluntary active euthanasia," was published in the *Journal of the American Medical Association* 1997; 278:2099–2104. Most of the case material was presented in a paper written with Barbara Coombs-Lee and Sally Nunn titled

"Palliative options of last resort: choosing the least harmful alternative" published in the *Annals of Internal Medicine* 2000; 132:488–493 as part of the University of Pennsylvania Center for Bioethics' "Finding Common Ground Project" Assisted Suicide Consensus Panel. The synthesis of material, subsequent editing, and added material is my responsibility alone.

References

1. Miller FG, Meier DE. Voluntary death: A comparison of terminal dehydration and physician-assisted suicide. *Ann Intern Med* 1998; 128:559–562.
2. Quill TE, Byock I. Responding to intractable terminal suffering: the role of terminal sedation and voluntary refusal of food and fluids. ACP-ASIM End-of-Life Care Consensus Panel. *Ann Intern Med* 2000; 132:408–414.
3. Cherny NI, Portenoy RK. Sedation in the management of refractory symptoms: Guidelines for evaluation and treatment. *J Palliat Care* 1994; 10:31–38.
4. Alpers A, Lo B. Physician-assisted suicide in Oregon: A bold experiment. *JAMA* 1995; 274:483–487.
5. Meier DE, Emmons C, Wallenstein S, Quill TE, Morrison RS, Cassel CK. A national survey of physician-assisted suicide and euthanasia in the United States. *N Engl J Med* 1998; 338:1193–1201.
6. Back AL, Wallace JI, Starks HE, Pearlman RA. Physician-assisted suicide and euthanasia in Washington State: Patient requests and physician responses. *JAMA* 1996; 275:919–925.
7. *Vacco v. Quill.* 1997. 117 S.Ct. 2293.
8. *Washington v. Glucksberg.* 1997. 117 S.Ct 2258.
9. Foley KM. Competent care for the dying instead of physician-assisted suicide. *N Engl J Med* 1997; 336:54–58.
10. American Board of Internal Medicine. Evaluation of humanistic qualities in the internist. *Ann Intern Med* 1983; 99:720–724.
11. American Board of Internal Medicine Committee. *Caring for the Dying: Identification and Promotion of Physician Competency.* 1–100. 1996. Philadelphia: American Board of Internal Medicine.
12. American Medical Association's Council on Ethical and Judicial Affairs. Decisions near the end of life. *JAMA* 1992; 276:2229–2233.
13. Fried C. *Right and Wrong.* Cambridge, Mass.: Harvard University Press, 1978.
14. Foley KM. Pain, physician-assisted suicide, and euthanasia. *Pain Forum* 1995; 4:163–178.
15. Quill TE. *Death and Dignity: Making Choices and Taking Charge.* New York: W.W. Norton and Co., 1993.
16. Quill TE. Principle of double effect and end-of-life pain management: Additional myths and a limited role. *J Palliat Med* 1998; 2:333–336.
17. Quill TE, Dresser R, Brock DW. Rule of double effect: A critique of its role in end-of-life decision making. *N Engl J Med* 1997; 337:1768–1771.
18. Meisel A. Legal myths about terminating life support. *Arch Intern Med* 1999; 151:1497–1502.
19. Miller DK, Coe RM, Hyers TM. Achieving consensus on withdrawing or withholding care for critically ill patients. *J Gen Intern Med* 1992; 7:475–480.

20. Brody H, Campbell ML, Faber-Langendoen K, Ogle KS. Withdrawing intensive life-sustaining treatment—recommendations for compassionate clinical management. *N Engl J Med* 1997; 336:652–657.
21. Weir RF, Gostin LO. Decisions to abate life-sustaining treatment for nonautonomous patients: Ethical standards and legal liability for physicians after Cruzan. *JAMA* 1990; 264:1846–1853.
22. Wilson WC, Smedira NG, Fink C, McDowell JA, Luce JM. Ordering and administration of sedatives and analgesics during the withholding and withdrawal of life support from critically ill patients. *JAMA* 1992; 267:949–953.
23. Eddy DM. A conversation with my mother. *JAMA* 1994; 272:179–181.
24. McCann RM, Hall WJ, Groth-Juncker A. Comfort care for terminally ill patients: the appropriate use of nutrition and hydration. *JAMA* 1994; 272:1263–1266.
25. Bernat JL, Gert B, Mogielnicki RP. Patient refusal of hydration and nutrition: An alternative to physician-assisted suicide or voluntary active euthanasia. *Arch Intern Med* 1993; 153:2723–2727.
26. Printz LA. Terminal dehydration, a compassionate treatment. *Arch Intern Med* 1992; 152:697–700.
27. Troug RD, Berde DB, Mitchell C, Grier HE. Barbiturates in the care of the terminally ill. *N Engl J Med* 1991; 327:1678–1682.
28. The history of intention in ethics. In: Kenny AJP, editor. *Anatomy of the Soul.* Oxford, England: Basil Blackwell, 1973; Appendix.
29. Saunders C, Sykes N. *The Management of Terminal Malignant Disease*, 3rd ed. London: Hoder Headline Group, 1993.
30. Coyle N, Adelhardt J, Foley KM, Portenoy RK. Character of terminal illness in the advanced cancer patient: Pain and other symptoms during the last four weeks of life. *J Pain Symptom Manage* 1990; 5:83–93.
31. Ingham J, Portenoy R. Symptom assessment. *Hematol Oncol Clin North Am* 1996; 10:21–39.
32. Mangan JT. An historical analysis of the principle of double effect. *Theol Studies* 1949; 10:41–61.
33. Ventafridda V, Ripamonti C, DeConno F, Tamburini M, Cassileth BR. Symptom prevalence and control during cancer patients' last days of life. *J Palliat Care* 1990; 6:7–11.
34. Brody H. Causing, intending and assisting death. *J Clin Ethics* 1993; 4:112–117.
35. Billings JA, Block SD. Slow euthanasia. *J Palliat Care* 1996; 12:21–30.
36. Orentlicher D. The Supreme Court and physician-assisted suicide—rejecting assisted suicide but embracing euthanasia. *N Engl J Med* 1997; 337:1236–1239.
37. *Evangelium Vitae.* 95 a.d.; Washington, D.C.: U.S. Catholic Conference, 1995.
38. Granfield D. *The Abortion Decision.* Garden City, NY: Image Books, 1971.
39. Garcia JLA. Double effect. In: Reich WT, editor. *Encyclopedia of Bioethics.* New York: Simon and Schuster, 1995, pp. 636–641.
40. Brock DW. Voluntary active euthanasia. *Hastings Cent Rep* 1992; 10–22.
41. Quill TE. Death and dignity: A case of individualized decision making. *N Engl J Med* 1991; 324:691–694.
42. Kane RL, Bernstein L, Wales J, Rothenberg R. Hospice effectiveness in controlling pain. *JAMA* 1985; 253:2683–2686.
43. Cohen JS, Fihn SD, Boyko EJ, Jonsen AR, Wood RW. Attitudes toward assisted suicide and euthanasia among physicains in Washington State. *N Engl J Med* 1994; 331:89–94.

44. Bachman JG, Alchser KH, Doukas DJ, Lichtenstein RL, Corning AD, Brody H. Attitudes of Michigan physicians and the public toward legalizing physician-assisted suicide and voluntary euthanasia. *N Engl J Med* 1996; 334:303–309.

45. Duberstein PR, Conwell Y, Cox C, Podgorski CA, Glazer RS, Caine ED. Attitudes toward self-determined death: A survey of primary care physicians. *J Am Geriatr Soc* 1995; 43:395–400.

46. Preston TA, Mero R. Observations concerning terminally ill patients who choose suicide. *J Pharm Care Pain Sympt Control* 1996; 1(183):192.

47. Groenewoud JH, van der Heide A, Onwuteaka-Philipsen BD, Willems DL, van der Maas PJ, van der Wal G. Clinical problems with the performance of euthanasia and physician-assisted suicide in the Netherlands. *N Engl J Med* 2000; 342:551–556.

48. Admiraal PV. Toepassing van euthanatica (The use of euthanatics). *Ned Tijdschr Geneeskd* 1995; 139:265–268.

49. Gaylin W, Kass LR, Pellegrino ED, Siegler M. "Doctors must not kill." *JAMA* 1988; 259:2139–2140.

50. Teno J, Lynn J. Voluntary active euthanasia: The individual case and public policy. *J Am Geriatr Soc* 1991; 39:827–830.

51. Kamisar Y. Some nonreligious views against proposed "mercy-killing" legislation. In: Leiser BM, editor. *Values in Conflict*. New York: MacMillan, 1981, pp. 109–121.

52. de Wachter MAM. Active euthanasia in the Netherlands. *JAMA* 1989; 262:3316–3319.

53. van der Maas PJ, van Delden JJM, Pijnenborg L. The Remmelink Study. *Health Policy* 1992.

54. van der Maas PJ, van der Wal G, Haverkate I, de Graaff CL, Kester JG, Onwuteaka-Philipsen BD, et al. Euthanasia, physician-assisted suicide, and other medical practices involving the end of life in the Netherlands, 1990–1995. *N Engl J Med* 1996; 335:1699–1705.

55. Hill CS Jr. When will adequate pain treatment be the norm? *JAMA* 1995; 274:1881–1882.

56. Quill TE. The ambiguity of clinical intentions. *N Engl J Med* 1993; 329:1039–1040.

57. Battin MP. *The Least Worst Death. Essays in Bioethics on the End of Life*. New York: Oxford University Press, 1994.

58. President's Commission for the Study of Ethical Problems in Medicine and Bio-medical and Behavioral Research. *Deciding to forgo life-sustaining treatment: A report on the ethical, medical and legal issues in treatment decisions*. Washington, DC: United States Government Printing Office, 1983.

59. Hastings Center. Guidelines on the Termination of Life-Sustaining Treatment and the Care of the Dying. 1987. New York: The Hastings Center.

60. Marquis DB. Four versions of the double effect. *J Med Philos* 1991; 16:515–544.

61. Kamm F. The doctrine of double effect: Reflections on theoretical and practical issues. *J Med Philos* 1991; 16:571–585.

62. Annas GJ. The promised end—constitutional aspects of physician-assisted suicide. *N Engl J Med* 1996; 335:683–687.

63. Beauchamp TL, Childress JF. *Principles of Biomedical Ethics*. New York: Oxford University Press, 1994.

64. Edwards MJ, Tolle SW. Disconnecting a ventilator at the request of a patient who knows he will then die: The doctor's anguish. *Ann Intern Med* 1992; 117:254–256.

65. Alpers A, Lo B. Does it make clinical sense to equate terminally ill patients who require life-sustaining interventions with those who do not? *JAMA* 1997; 277:1705–1708.

66. Orentlicher D. The legalization of physician-assisted suicide. *N Engl J Med* 1996; 335:663–667.
67. American Law Institute. (1985). Model Penal Code and Commentaries. Section 2.02 ed. Philadelphia: American Law Institute.
68. Quill TE, Brody RV. "You promised me I wouldn't die like this." A bad death as a medical emergency. *Arch Intern Med* 1995; 155:1250–1254.
69. Welie JVM. The medical exception: Physicians, euthanasia and the Dutch criminal law. *J Med Philos* 1992; 17:419–437.
70. Quill TE, Cassel CK. Nonabandonment: A central obligation for physicians. *Ann Intern Med* 1995; 122:368–374.
71. Boston L, Weir FR. Life and death choices after Cruzan: Case law and standards of professional conduct. *Milbank Q* 1991; 69:143–173.
72. Buchanan A, Brock D. *Deciding for Others: The Ethics of Surrogate Decision Making*. Cambridge: Cambridge University Press, 1989.
73. Sulmasy DP, Terry PB, Weisman CS, Miller DJ, Stallings RY, Vettese MA, Haller KB. The accuracy of substituted judgments in patients with terminal diagnoses. *Ann Intern Med* 1998; 128:621–629.
74. Kuczewski MG. Reconceiving the family. The process of consent in medical decision-making. *Hastings Cent Rep* 1996; 26:30–37.
75. Brock D. What is the moral authority of family members to act as surrogates for incompetent patients? *Milbank Q* 1996; 74:599–618.
76. Karlawish JH, Quill TE, Meier DE. A consensus-based approach to providing palliative care to patients who lack decision-making capacity. ACP-ASIM End-of-Life Care Consensus Panel. *Ann Intern Med* 1999; 130:835–840.
77. Quill TE, Cassel CK, Meier DE. Care of the hopelessly ill. Proposed criteria for physician-assisted suicide. *N Engl J Med* 1992; 327:1380–1384.
78. Brody H. Assisted death—A compassionate response to a medical failure. *N Engl J Med* 1992; 327:1384–1385.
79. Miller FG, Quill TE, Brody H, Fletcher JC, Gostin LO, Meier DE. Regulating physician-assisted death. *N Engl J Med* 1994; 331:119–123.
80. Baron CH, Bergstresser C, Brock DW, Cole GF, Dorfman NS, Johnson JA, et al. Statute: A model state act to authorize and regulate physician-assisted suicide. *Harvard Journal on Legislation* 1996; 33:1–34.
81. Cantor NL, Thomas GC. Pain relief, acceleration of death, and criminal law. *Kennedy Inst Ethics J* 1996; 6:107–127.
82. Quill TE. *A Midwife Through the Dying Process. Stories of Healing and Hard Choices at the End of Life*. Baltimore: Johns Hopkins University Press, 1996.
83. Aries P. *The Hour of Our Death*. New York: Oxford University Press, 1991.
84. Singer PA, Siegler M. Euthanasia—a critique. *N Engl J Med* 1975; 292:78–80.
85. Foley KM. The treatment of cancer pain. *N Engl J Med* 1989; 313:84–95.
86. Loxterkamp D. A good death is hard to find: Preliminary reports of a hospice doctor. *J Am Board Fam Pract* 1993; 6:415–417.

13

End-of-Life Care in the Netherlands and the United States: A Comparison of Values, Justifications, and Practices

Voluntary active euthanasia (VAE) and physician-assisted suicide (PAS) remain technically illegal in the Netherlands, but the practices are openly tolerated provided that physicians adhere to carefully constructed guidelines.[1-4] Harsh criticism by authors in the United States[5-7] and Great Britain[8] has made achieving a balanced understanding of the clinical, moral, and policy implications of this Dutch practice very difficult. Similar practice patterns probably exist in the United States,[9-12] but outside of Oregon they are conducted in secret because of a more uncertain legal and ethical climate. In this chapter, end-of-life care in the United States and the Netherlands is compared with regard to underlying values, justifications, and practices. The risks and benefits of each system for a real patient who is faced with a common end-of-life clinical dilemma are explored. The chapter closes with a description of the challenges for public policy makers in both countries.

An earlier version of this chapter was published in collaboration with Gerrit Kimsma, a Dutch physician, in the *Cambridge Quarterly of Healthcare Ethics* 1997;6:189–204. The additions and editing from the original manuscript are solely my opinion

Background

The underlying legal, clinical, professional, and attitudinal characteristics of the Netherlands with respect to end-of-life public policy have been reviewed elsewhere.[1,2,13–16] The Dutch acute care system utilizes all modern technologies, and virtually all Dutch citizens have comprehensive health insurance that includes nursing home care if necessary. VAE and PAS have been openly discussed and practiced since the courts ruled leniently on the first prosecuted case in 1973.[1] Although the practices remain technically illegal, they now have wide social acceptance, supported by case law, several state commissions, medical and legal professional societies, and legislation. Physicians can feel confident that they will not be prosecuted provided they adhere to clearly publicized criteria.[15] Patients can feel confident that their doctors will not be afraid to act if their suffering becomes overwhelming. The Netherlands is the only country in the world where end-of-life practices have been comprehensively studied through a government-sponsored commission.[16,17] Discussion about end-of-life suffering is sophisticated and wide-ranging in the Netherlands; the notion that suffering sometimes is a much bigger enemy than death has wide public acceptance.

In addition to coverage for hospitalization and long-term care, the Dutch have a model system of primary care, with equitable distribution throughout the country. Dutch primary care physicians (*huisarts*) generally live and practice in the same neighborhood for their entire careers, so long-term relationships with patients are the rule rather than the exception. The Dutch have been criticized, however, for not having adequate hospice care, and for turning to VAE too quickly.[5–7] Most Dutch policy makers argue that palliative care is being adequately done within their existing systems of care. Many of the existing volunteer-based Dutch hospices are underutilized. Dutch citizens tend to be skeptical about hospice's religious roots, manifest by its blanket opposition to VAE no matter how severe the patient's suffering. Most religiously affiliated Dutch hospices remain morally opposed to VAE under any circumstances. However, secular hospice workers in the Netherlands acknowledge that VAE might be necessary for "a few" patients who fail hospice care, and they see the practices as complementary rather than mutually exclusive.

Dutch physicians are committed conceptually to palliative care, but training and practice patterns have lagged behind that commitment. Attempts to close this gap are under way. Family physicians are now being explicitly taught to consider VAE as only one option within a program of palliative care for terminal patients.[18] Physicians providing second opinions in VAE cases now must be "independent" from the primary physician (i.e., not in the same practice group), but there is still no requirement that such physicians have expertise in palliative care. A small network of volunteer hospices is growing, and policy makers increasingly recognize that palliative care in the Netherlands is not guided by a comprehensive, system-wide plan. A university professorship in palliative care has been established in Rotterdam, and several experiments for residential hospice care have been funded by the government. Since excellent palliative care is the standard of care for the dying, exceptional interventions like VAE and PAS make sense only in the context of its widespread availability.[19–21] Unfortunately, organized palliative care remains a weak link in an otherwise exemplary health care system in the Netherlands, with too little training for all physicians, too few palliative care experts, and no organized system for handling palliative care emergencies and reimbursement.

The United States has the most expensive health care system in the world, yet approximately 43 million citizens remain uninsured. At the same time, evidence of overtreatment at the end of life, often against the wishes of the patient and family, continues to be found.[22] The United States trains many physicians, but they are not equitably distributed.[23] Few medical schools and residency training programs have comprehensive curricula in palliative care,[24,25] though this deficiency is gradually improving. An aggressive effort to get overall medical spending under control is under way—primarily through large, capitated health care systems that manage primary care, in-hospital care, and long-term care—but such systems so far appear to be driven mainly by cost containment rather than principles of quality and universal access.[26]

The United States has a well-organized system of Medicare-funded hospice programs available in most large population centers.[27,28] These programs use a multidisciplinary team to reinforce and support care given by families in the patient's own home. Most also have access to residential facilities for palliative care emergencies. The Medicare hospice benefit has now been extended to residents of nursing homes and small, privately run residential hospice houses. Hospice costs are paid on a fixed, per diem basis. The availability of hospice has increased dramatically in the last ten years, yet it continues to be underutilized in the United States as compared to continuing futile aggressive care toward the end of life.[29] Hospice referrals are often made very late in patients' illnesses, if at all, depriving patients and families of the full range of available services. Furthermore, hospice benefits are mainly available to patients with cancer who are likely to die within six months. Formal hospice programs are currently unavailable to the majority of patients who are dying of chronic degenerative diseases of the lungs, heart, and nervous systems whose prognoses are more uncertain and who may want to continue at least some aggressive disease directed therapies.[30] Hospice in the United States has organizationally been opposed to VAE and PAS, arguing that "virtually all" palliative care problems can be solved by other means.[31] However, there is considerable diversity of opinion within its ranks about the place of these practices as a last resort in the small number of cases where palliative care becomes ineffective or inadequate.

VAE remains illegal everywhere in the United States, and is likely to be vigorously prosecuted if uncovered. PAS, on the other hand, is in legal flux: It has been formally legalized in the state of Oregon after two referenda and multiple legal challenges.[32] PAS is illegal in most other states. An "Oregon-like" referendum was narrowly defeated in Maine in the fall of 2000, and a state-based constitutional challenge is under way in Alaska. In 1997, the United States Supreme Court ruled that that there was no constitutionally protected right to PAS, but it also gave a green light to state-based experiments with legalization.[33,34] Although PAS remains illegal in most jurisdictions in the United States, the practice is usually not prosecuted if uncovered, provided it remains undetected by the media.[35–37] Public opinion polls show that approximately two-thirds of the public favor doctors being able to actively ease death, although more hesitation is expressed at the voting booths when the legalization of PAS is considered, with an almost 50–50 split in Washington, California, and Oregon, and Maine.[9,38–41] The public debate in the United States has been loud and polarized, with little willingness to explore common ground or to creatively look for new solutions that might better meet the needs of dying patients.

Values

Autonomy and individual freedom are highly valued and have long traditions in both the Netherlands and the United States.[13,14] The fundamental importance of these concepts for morality is respecting the beliefs and convictions of others.[42–45] Individuals from both countries demand a central voice in all aspects of their lives, and in particular in their medical care. Patients have the legal right to be fully informed about, and then consent to or refuse, medical treatments, rather than depending entirely on the recommendations of their doctors. The Dutch may have more trust in physicians, based on long-term relationships, and therefore more acceptance of paternalistic aspects of medical care, but both cultures agree in theory that a patient's autonomous, fully informed choices should guide all important medical decisions.

The Netherlands has a strong tradition of tolerance for individual expression, as long as it does not seriously infringe upon the rights of others.[1,2] In addition to policies that allow individuals a wide range of options at the end of life, Dutch society openly tolerates "soft" drugs (marijuana), prostitution, abortion, and homosexuality. Despite easy access, the Netherlands has one of the lowest abortion rates in the world, in part because the Dutch combine this "tolerant" policy with comprehensive, obligatory educational and outreach programs about birth control and family planning. Tolerance is found among most religious groups, who may disagree with certain policies in principle but are less inclined to try to impose their views on others. The media takes its public role in debating controversial issues seriously, but is less prone than U.S. media to sensationalism and tends to give less voice to the extremes. Dutch problem solving tends to favor consensus building and negotiation more than discussion and confrontation. The Dutch legal system, which is civil rather than common as in the United States, tends to be more tolerant and less punitive. Legal decisions are in the hands of judges rather than juries, sentences are often symbolic, and jail terms are infrequent and relatively short. There is little malpractice litigation, and little or no added compensation for pain and suffering.

The United States tends to be both intolerant and punitive in similar domains. Pro-life religious groups are well organized, politically active, and willing to impose their views on others. Access to safe abortions is becoming more legally restricted, and those providing this service often do so at considerable personal risk.[46] At the same time, teenage pregnancy has reached epidemic proportions, and education about and access to effective birth control are being contentiously opposed. Despite widespread use of soft drugs, legalization is too controversial politically to be seriously considered. The percent of the population in jail is rapidly increasing in the United States, a vivid symbol of the tendency to try to control social behavior through punishment and fear. The media fuel intolerance by favoring sound bites over substance, and giving disproportionate coverage to the loudest, most extreme voices on either side of a debate. A sophisticated public discussion about end-of-life care is very difficult to conduct in this environment.

The individual's obligation to contribute to a greater good is well developed in the Netherlands, and is captured in the concept of "solidarity," meaning roughly that the state has a responsibility to protect the rights and interests of the less fortunate.[13,14] All Dutch residents pay toward funds that guarantee universal access to health insurance covering primary care, hospitalization, and nursing home care. When compared to the United States, the Dutch are more highly taxed, have a larger middle class, and have a narrower gap between rich and poor. The Netherlands, the size of Rhode Island with a population of 15 million, is a much smaller and more homogeneous country than the United States. Achieving consensus on potentially divisive social issues has been a condition for survival, and may therefore be more culturally ingrained. Furthermore, the Netherlands has a tradition of coalition governments, because no single party can gain a parliamentary majority and rule single-handedly. Overall, the societal commitment to solidarity provides a balancing force for the emphasis on individual autonomy.

In the United States, the rights of the individual are seen as more important than those of the larger community. This imbalance has become even more exaggerated by current political forces in Washington, D.C., constantly emphasizing the individual's responsibility for his own survival and the moral inferiority of the less fortunate. The basic safety net upon which vulnerable populations depend is under vigorous attack, while the rights of the most fortunate are being strengthened. Whereas the U.S. health care system is being creatively reinvented, the main motivation is cost control, and there is little principled discussion about how to improve access to health care for the 43 million citizens who are currently uninsured.[26] The notion that all citizens would pay for guaranteed universal access to basic health care, much less long-term care, has become politically unachievable. The United States is so large geographically, and so diverse culturally, that achieving a strong moral sense of community and solidarity is one of its greatest challenges.

Finally, the Dutch are very pragmatic.[2,14] They try to solve difficult problems and achieve practical solutions, even if it requires compromise. Dutch legislators and citizens are willing to try policies that are imperfect, and even internally inconsistent, in order to address an important problem. For example, keeping VAE and PAS illegal but at the same time developing explicit criteria to cover circumstances when they will not be prosecuted is a characteristic compromise.[1,2,14] It allows a controversial practice because of a compelling perceived need, but also maintains legal oversight and expresses societal ambivalence. Although this solution is far from ideal, the Dutch are willing to let the practice evolve until a better answer is found, rather than prohibit the practices entirely, or force them underground because the policy issues are too complex and difficult. The downside of this willingness to compromise is that public debate sometimes lacks sharpness, and important differences and nuances are sometimes prematurely glossed over.

Pragmatism is frequently lacking in the United States. Public debates tend to be polarized, and compromise is equated with weakness. The constant glare of the media forces policy makers to frame issues according to superficial public appeal, rather than openly explore the depths and nuances of complex social problems. The middle ground frequently gets lost in the rhetoric and competition. Individuals are forced to choose between being "pro choice" and "pro life," while most of the population want policies to both favor life and allow choice. Public debates tend to be "win-lose" and "either-or," giving a disproportionately loud voice to the political extremes. Practical solutions frequently get lost in the posturing. Exploration of the edges of a topic can sometimes clarify issues during debate, but this can also lead to principle-based, all-or-none solutions that serve no one particularly well.

In summary, some of the contrasting values observed in the Netherlands and the United States can be explained by the differences in countries' size, cultural diversity, and economic disparity. Yet there are common traditions in both countries that favor individual autonomy, and striking differences in traditions of tolerance, solidarity, and pragmatism in reacting to threats to health, social stability, and justice, that may in part explain different public policy approaches to end-of-life decision making.

Justification Used for End-of-Life Decision Making

In the United States, as discussed in Chapter 11, the rule of double effect is often employed in moral reasoning at the end of life.[47-50] This concept, derived from Catholic tradition, relies on a rigid distinction between consequences that are intended and those that are unintended. Intentionally causing death is always evil, no matter how terrible the patient's clinical circumstances. However, if clinicians intervene with the intent to relieve suffering, and the patient dies as an unintended consequence, the latter is a tolerated "double effect." Death may even be foreseen as a potential conse-quence by the physician and wished for by a patient, but it cannot be even partially intended by the physician if the intervention is to remain within the confines of the rule of double effect.

Most Dutch physicians reject the principle of double effect when applied to clinical decision making, viewing it as a religious concept that is in-adequate to cover complex end-of-life decisions.[51] The Dutch are taught to take responsibility for both intended and unintended consequences, and the notion that a clearly foreseen consequence that is not intended could be free of moral culpability is felt to be psychologically and morally problematic. The physician's potentially active, conscious role in easing death in the face of unbearable suffering is not morally rejected out of hand. Most Dutch physi-cians believe their primary responsibility is to ease suffering, and that extreme, unrelievable suffering of a terminally ill patient is a sufficiently grave reason for allowing extraordinary interventions like VAE or PAS.[1,2] In lieu of relying on "active" versus "passive" or "intended" versus "unintended" distinctions, the Dutch have developed more descriptive categories for end-of-life practices:[16] *(1)* acts intending to alleviate pain and suffering, *(2)*nontreatment decisions, *(3)* voluntary active euthanasia and physician-assisted suicide, and *(4)* life-ending acts without explicit request. This redefinition allows the specific moral prob-lems inherent in each area to be more objectively explored rather than obfus-cated by abstract, imprecise terminology. Not responding to a dying patient who is suffering unbearably and wanting to die because of abstract categorical distinctions would be unacceptable to most Dutch physicians.

In the Netherlands, a secular legal concept called *force majeure* guides decision making about VAE and PAS.[52,53] *Force majeure* covers "situations of necessity" where the physician's duties to preserve life and to relieve suffering come into conflict. The concept was employed by the highest Dutch judicial authority, the High Council, in 1984, eleven years after the first case was tried.

The judge in the first case in 1973 based his legal decision on expert medical testimony, stating that no physician should be expected to continue to "prolong life to the bitter end."[54] At the end of life, the duty to relieve suffering outweighs the duty to preserve life. Under circumstances where a patient wants to die because his or her suffering is unbearable, the physician's moral obligation to the patient as a caregiver outweighs any duty to obey the law as a citizen. VAE and PAS technically remain crimes, but under specified circumstances they are not punishable. The actor is either not prosecuted, or, if tried and found guilty, not punished, provided the clinical circumstances warrant the exception. The exceptional circumstances have been legally codified so doctors now know they will not be punished if all agreed-upon criteria have been satisfied.[15] The practices of PAS and VAE are supported by a large majority of the public and the medical profession, although formal legalization of the practices has yet to be completed.*

Reporting cases of VAE and PAS has increased since the legal requirements of *force majeure* were agreed upon, but the rate is still at only about 50%.[17] Under-reporting may partially reflect physicians' unwillingness to admit to murder for what they view as a compassionate act. Other physicians may not want to expose themselves and their patients' families to judicial review. Some unreported cases probably do not meet all of the agreed-upon criteria, and therefore might be subject to a lengthy trial process and potential conviction. *Force majeure* is used to justify "usual" cases that meet all agreed-upon criteria, but the courts repeatedly rely on the same reasoning to cover truly exceptional cases when some of the criteria are not fully met.[55] Limits to the practice of VAE are being explored in the Netherlands, including pure psychological suffering, incurable but not imminently terminal illness, and how to treat extreme suffering when a patient loses the mental capacity to consent at the very end. *Force majeure* appears to be a blunt legal instrument that does not easily discriminate among these circumstances. Recently, some Dutch lawyers have openly questioned the suitability of the law to judge these complex medical issues, and have suggested it may be appropriate for physicians and policy makers to seek a consensus after more reflection and study.

Comparison of How Death Is Eased

Other than documentation of overly aggressive treatment at the end of life[22] and reports about legalized physician-assisted suicide in Oregon over the last two years,[11,12] there are few reliable epidemiologic studies about how doctors participate in their patients' deaths in the United States. The punitive legal

---

* After passage by the Dutch legislature, in the fall of 2000, formal legalization is anticipated in 2001.

and ethical environment, combined with constant, exaggerating glare from the media, make it difficult to reliably ascertain such information. In theory, however, there is agreement about several categories of end-of-life practices.

As explored in Chapter 12, withholding and withdrawing life-sustaining treatment and aggressive symptom management have wide acceptance in the United States. How frequently death is consciously eased with these practices is unknown. About 10%–15% of kidney failure patients on dialysis die because they choose to stop treatment,[56,57] though there is substantial variation between dialysis centers. There are some data that patients' and families' willingness to stop life supports is increasing in the United States,[58] but how much this reflects initial over-use or potential under-use is impossible to discern.

Terminal sedation (TS) and voluntarily stopping eating and drinking (VSED) also have legal support, but how available they are in practice is unknown. The use of TS for patients in hospice programs varies from 0% to 50% of deaths, suggesting an uneven access to the practice owing more to the attitudes and values of practitioners than to those of patients.[59–61] There are no reliable reported data about the frequency of VSED.

Outside the state of Oregon, PAS is passively prohibited but secretly practiced in the United States. A recent survey of Washington State physicians showed that 12% had received a genuine request for PAS within the year studied, and 24% responded by providing a potentially lethal prescription.[9] Another 4% of physicians received requests for VAE, and 24% of those provided a lethal injection. A national survey with elaborate protections of anonymity showed similar freqencies.[10] Currently Oregon is the only state in the country that allows legal access to physician-assisted suicide, subject to the carefully constructed requirements outlined in Table 13-1. Of note are the restriction of the practice to competent, terminally ill patients, the 15 day waiting period between initial request and access to the medication, and the requirement of a second opinion on all criteria.

The first two years of data about the legal practice of PAS in Oregon have now been reported.[11,12] In total, only 27 patients died from PAS in 1999 and 16 in 1998, representing less than 0.1% of total deaths in each year. All of the patients had health insurance, most were highly educated, most were on hospice programs and all had access to such programs, all were Caucasian, and the median age was over 70. Metastatic cancer was the most common diagnosis, followed by amyotrophic lateral sclerosis and chronic obstructive lung disease. Uncontrolled pain was rarely the dominant reason cited by physicians or family members for this decision, and none cited financial concerns. More commonly, the reasons cited by patients as reported by physicians and family members were a combination of loss of control of bodily functions, loss of autonomy, an inability to participate in activities that make life enjoyable, and a determination to control the manner of death. Since PAS has

TABLE 13–1. Legal Requirements for Physician-Assisted Suicide in Oregon: The Oregon Death with Dignity Act

General Patient Requirements for Making a Legal Request

Adult 18 years or older

Resident of Oregon

Mentally capable of making health care decisions

Terminal illness (lead to death within 6 months)

Procedural Requirements for Responding to Legal Requests

Patient provides
- two verbal requests separated by at least 15 days
- written, witnessed request

Prescribing physician and consulting physician must
- confirm diagnosis and prognosis
- determine the patient's mental capacity
- arrange for psychological examination if doubt about capacity

Prescribing physician must
- inform patient about alternatives (hospice, pain control)
- request (but not require) that next of kin be notified

been legalized in Oregon, hospice referrals have increased by approximately 20%; morphine prescriptions per capita have increased, making Oregon one of the highest rates in the nation; and in-hospital deaths are the lowest in the nation when compared to at-home deaths.[62,63] Rather than undermining end-of-life care, the first two years of data from Oregon suggest that it is associated with improvements in all of the facets studied, and there has been no evidence of abuse or over-use.

In addition to the infrequent practice of PAS in the United States, some physicians probably learn to hide their actions and intentions within the inherent ambiguity of double effect, treating terminal symptoms very aggressively when suffering is severe and a patient wants to die.[51,64] Given a volatile, punitive environment where intentionally easing death is expressly forbidden,[6,7] they may find it safer to hedge their intentions or even to turn their backs on patients with severe suffering, rather than risk being second-guessed and subject to highly politicized professional and legal reviews.[65]

The treatment of patients in the United States who lose the ability to speak for themselves is also epidemiologically unexplored.[66] In practice, the presumption to treat in the presence of uncertainty often leads to over-use of aggressive medical technology on those who are dying and have become cognitively incapacitated.[22] We know very little about how death is eased when suffering is severe with these patients. Presumably, aggressive symptom-relieving measures are used in accordance with the doctrine of double effect, life-sustaining treatments are stopped, and TS is offered as a last resort for severe suffering that cannot otherwise be relieved. Unfortunately, little is known and honest discussion is risky and rare among physicians, making access to these practices erratic and uneven at best.

In the Netherlands, VAE and PAS are openly practiced subject to safeguards (outlined in Table 13–2).[2] Substantive safeguards require that patient decisions be voluntary and fully informed, suffering be unbearable, and that there be no reasonable alternatives. Procedural requirements include obtaining an independent second opinion, reporting to legal authorities, and documenting the process in the patient's medical record. Additional professional obligations include the proper dosing of medications and availability to respond to complications. Substantive and professional requirements are perceived to be more important than procedural safeguards, and there is a strong moral sense within the profession that the patient's unique suffering must be responded to no matter what the legal requirements.

The Netherlands is the only country in the world where end-of-life practices have been scrutinized epidemiologically. According to the Remmelink Reports,[16,17] "nontreatment decisions" (equivalent to stopping or not starting life supports) and "alleviating pain and suffering" (equivalent to aggressive pain management) each account for about 17.5% of deaths. VAE accounts for 1.8%–2.4% of all deaths, and PAS another 0.2%–0.4%. In 0.7%–0.8% of deaths, a "life-ending act without explicit consent" was performed on incapacitated

TABLE 13–2. Dutch Safeguards for Voluntary Active Euthanasia and Physician-assisted Suicide

Substantive Safeguards

Decision voluntary and fully informed

Suffering unbearable

No reasonable alternatives

Procedural Requirements

Independent second opinion

Reporting to legal authorities

Documentation in patient's medical record

Professional Obligations

Proper dosing of medications

Availability to respond to complications

patients, raising concern about whether guidelines restricting VAE to competent patients can be enforced in practice.[55] There was no separate coding for practices like TS in the Remmelink studies, which is how palliative care physicians in the United States deal with severe suffering in incapacitated patients. The Dutch view TS as a form of "slow euthanasia," and would probably therefore code such practices and clinical situations as forms of "life-ending acts without explicit consent."

The Remmelink Reports provided ammunition for both sides of the debate in the United States. Those favoring a more open practice cite the following:

1. The incidence of VAE (1.8%–2.4%) and PAS (0.2%–0.4%) were low compared to alleviating pain and suffering (17.5%) and nontreatment decisions (17.5%) as a percentage of overall deaths.
2. The number of inquiries about VAE was high (25,000) compared to genuine requests (9,000) and acts (2,700), suggesting a complex process of reassurance, assessment, and search for alternatives.
3. Unrelieved pain was the sole reason for the requests in only 5% of VAE and PAS cases. More often it was a complex mixture of loss of dignity (57%), unworthy dying (46%), dependency on others (33%), and being tired of life (23%), frequently in combination with pain (46%).
4. Relatively few VAE deaths were among nursing home residents (40/2,700).
5. Life was shortened by less than one week in 58% and less than one month in 83% of cases.
6. Practice patterns seemed relatively stable over the five years between the two reports, alleviating many concerns about the "slippery slope."
7. Reporting incidences of VAE and PAS to the legal authorities increased from 25% to 50% in the time between the two studies.

Opponents of sanctioning VAE or PAS focus on other aspects of the report:

1. There were 1,000 cases (0.7%–0.8%) of "life-ending acts without explicit request" by the patient. When a small subgroup of these cases was analyzed in detail, 59% were based on a prior discussion and commitment between doctor and patient, but in the remaining 41% no such discussion had occurred. In the latter group, most cases were based on extreme suffering, imminent death, requests by the family, and substituted judgment, but there were a few exceptions from the early 1980s that "should not have happened."[67]
2. Although the substantive guidelines were generally adhered to, only 28% of cases were reported to the legal authorities in 1991, and only 60% of

physicians kept written records. Since the criteria for prosecution have been clarified, the reporting rate has risen to 50%,[17] but it is still far from complete.

3. Because physicians' "partial intentions" were to end life in many cases where medicine was given to alleviate pain and suffering and in some non-treatment decisions, some commentators have argued that the real number of cases of VAE is closer to 20,000.[68] However, Dutch physicians may think about and express their intentions about similar acts differently from those for whom the double effect is a central moral and legal tenant.

Most Dutch physicians believe the number of "life-ending acts without explicit request" must be minimized, although many experienced physicians believe they cannot be totally eliminated without abandoning some incapacitated patients who suffer enormously at the very end. They also argue that these cases are currently being managed with TS in the United States, and that the practices are more similar than different. Most Dutch physicians believe that cases of VAE and PAS should be reported, but some find the reporting process burdensome and others resent having to admit to a serious crime for what they believe is a compassionate act. There has also been a highly publicized, troubling case of VAE of a psychiatric patient in the Netherlands.[69] Although the courts ruled that patients could not be discriminated against because their suffering was nonphysical, this case has generated serious clinical and policy discussion about how to set limits on the practice of VAE.

Case Report

A brief clinical presentation will illustrate both the potential benefits and the risks of the U.S. and Dutch systems to dying patients.

A 75 year-old man was diagnosed with metastatic adenocarcinoma. He had seen his wife die in pain, and then "out of her mind" from the side effects of high-dose pain medicines. He wanted to live as long as his life could remain meaningful, but he knew from the outset that he would rather die than be subjected to such suffering and humiliation as he had witnessed with his wife. He initially chose palliative chemotherapy, and had a good response that allowed him to remain active for the subsequent year. When his cancer recurred in his neck, he was treated with palliative radiation with excellent pain relief. He was referred to hospice at that time, and was promised that "he would not die alone or in pain."

In the Netherlands, a discussion between physician and patient might have started at this point on the specifics of the patient's ideas and expectations concerning death and dying. If this patient requested VAE at this early phase, no Dutch physician would feel an obligation to honor the request because intolerable suffering was not present. The presence of a well-considered, enduring request is one important requirement, but the physician also must find the request to be based on current suffering that is unbearable, not distorted by depression, and not relievable by other palliative measures. Agreeing with a patient that there are no other options left involves both an external process (determined by the law) and an internal one of acceptance by the physician (determined more by personal values and experience). Many patients request reassurance about the possibility of VAE in the future if suffering becomes extreme, but relatively few request the act itself. This particular patient would probably have found reassurance in the possibility of a physician-assisted death in his future, given his values and what he had witnessed with his wife. However, if he had been able to choose death at this point, he might have missed the opportunity to achieve a meaningful end to his life.

In the United States, a similar discussion about last-resort practices might have been initiated in response to his fears about dying as his wife had. If he had lived in Oregon, this discussion could have included the possibility of PAS in the future, but he would not have qualified at this early stage, again because of the absence of extreme suffering. Outside of Oregon, this line of inquiry would have been confounded by the illegality of the practice. Therefore, a physician's willingness to offer this possibility in the future would depend not only on his personal values but on his willingness to take a substantial legal and professional risk on the patient's behalf. The patient and physician might have also explored TS and VSED as last-resort options that could be legally offered, but again he would not have qualified for either practice at present, according to the guidelines offered in Table 12–4.

The patient entered a hospice program at this point, and all medical efforts were devoted to sustaining the quality of his remaining life. His three months in hospice included excellent symptom management, healing contact with his children from whom he had been estranged, and spiritual work to better understand his life and prepare for death. Both he and his family were immeasurably enriched by his experience. When his pain began to accelerate toward the very end, he had completed the work of preparation and was now ready for death. Rapid, systematic increases and alterations in his pain regimen did not bring his pain under control. The peace and readiness he and his family had achieved were being undermined, and replaced by fear and disintegration. At this point, he requested a physician-assisted death, which is not legally permitted in the United States.

In the Netherlands, he would now have met eligibility criteria, because he was competent and his suffering had become intolerable. He could have selected a time, said good-bye to his family, and died by an explicit act that would have been acceptable to him and his family. In Oregon, he would have had to request medication for PAS before the last minute because of the requisite 15 day waiting period. He probably would have qualified according to the other criteria summarized in Table 13–1, and all criteria would have been verified by a consultant. Outside of Oregon, any possibility of PAS would have been conducted in secret, without the benefit of a second opinion. A willing physician, it is hoped, would have assessed the patient's mental capacity, his severity of suffering, and the adequacy of palliative care, but there would have been no documentation and no assurance that all dimensions had been fully addressed. His physician could also have legally explored TS as a way to assist him in escaping suffering.

The patient was hospitalized as a palliative care emergency in order to more rapidly respond to his deteriorating situation. Intravenous analgesics were rapidly and systematically increased, and his pain was controlled within 12 hours. Unfortunately, he began hallucinating as a side effect of the analgesics. His pain was relieved, but he was now paranoid, "out of his mind," much as his wife had been before her death. Changing doses and analgesics, and using major and minor tranquilizers, did not resolve the problem. Palliative care and pain relief specialists were consulted. His family pressed for a solution, lamenting that this particular type of death was his worst nightmare. They very clearly and passionately articulated their belief that he would rather be dead than in such a state. Something had to be done. He could no longer give his consent, although all who knew him felt that would have been his wish. He was offered, through his daughter, who was acting as his proxy, the option of terminal sedation with barbiturates. He was sedated to unconsciousness, not given intravenous fluids, and then "allowed to die" of dehydration over the next five days.

Dying under the equivalent of general anesthesia (TS) was not a terrible death. Because the patient was unconscious, he was probably not suffering, but this patient would clearly have chosen an explicit act if it had been legally available. This particular act was driven by the law and by current ethical distinctions, not by his or his family's values. The moral differences between such "passive" acts that inevitably result in death and VAE or PAS are hazy at best, and both acts are subject to the similar risks of abuse to vulnerable populations. Several family members commented that we treat our animals better than we treat humans, for we would never sedate a dying animal to unconsciousness so that it would be "allowed to die" of dehydration. Dutch physicians who considered this case found it disturbing to subject patients to such a morally ambiguous process that they considered to be "slow euthanasia." If the patient's death had been eased in this manner in the Netherlands, he would have fallen under one of the troubling 1,000 involuntary cases, since the Dutch have no separate category for TS and do not see it as distinct morally or clinically from euthanasia. All directly involved in the case agreed that TS with barbiturates was an imperfect solution, but it was far better than allowing him to continue to suffer, out of his mind and passively waiting for death.

Challenges

The health care systems in the Netherlands and the United States have much in common, and many differences. The challenges in creating systems of care for the dying that are simultaneously caring, responsive, and safe are considerably different in each, driven in part by the values, justifications, and practices each country has chosen to emphasize in its public policies.

Comprehensive Palliative Care Is the Standard of Care for the Dying

In the Netherlands, there is a genuine conceptual commitment to palliative care as part of primary, hospital, and nursing home care. Yet formal hospice programs are largely voluntary and highly person dependent, and there is little enthusiasm for creating an additional separate system of care. Educational programs to improve the quality of palliative care are being developed, but relatively little time is devoted to the subject in the medical curriculum, and skill levels are variable. Beds need to be designated for palliative care emergencies, and expert consultants must be available to ensure that all palliative possibilities have been considered before VAE is performed. VAE and PAS make sense only in the context of excellent, comprehensive palliative care. It would be tragic for someone to choose VAE when suffering from symptoms that might have been relieved by available medical interventions.

The United States has an excellent system of hospice care, mainly for patients dying of cancer. However, 43 million citizens are without any health care insurance at all. Palliative care, as exemplified in hospice programs, is the standard of care for dying patients in the United States against which all other approaches must be measured. It uses the resources of a multidisciplinary team and volunteers to address the needs of dying patients and their families. U.S.

hospices are largely home based and dependent on family participation, but inpatient beds are also designated for palliative care emergencies. Palliative care programs need to be developed for patients stricken with the advanced stages of all chronic degenerative diseases, so that all dying patients have medically supported alternatives to continuing aggressive, technology-dominated care that has outlived its usefulness. Stopping life-sustaining therapy, TS, VSED, and PAS (if legal) should be considered only for those cases where palliative care has been found to be ineffective or unacceptable. Access to palliative care must always be a requirement before a physician-assisted death, no matter what category, is seriously considered—especially in the United States, where health care insurance coverage is so variable and inequitable. None of these practices must ever be substitutes for the best available medical care. Easing death in the face of unbearable suffering should not be too hard, too easy, or too arbitrary.

In the United States, many patients genuinely fear that their doctors will not help them to die, even if their suffering becomes overwhelming, humiliating, and not otherwise relievable. Easing death is too difficult in the United States, often arbitrarily dependent on the presence or absence of life supports, or on standards of intention that do not seem genuine or honest. The safest course legally for a physician whose patient's suffering becomes extreme is to under-medicate and even abandon. Since the dying of real persons rarely fits within idealized palliative care protocols, the United States needs to create an environment that ensures its doctors understand that their primary professional obligation is to act in solidarity with their dying patients and their families, rather than in fear of legal or professional recrimination.[70] Whereas the legal fears of physicians in the United States are probably exaggerated, they nevertheless exert a strong negative influence on the care of the dying.[71]

Dutch physicians are committed to responding to the individual situation of their dying patients, and most patients know they will not be abandoned if their suffering becomes overwhelming. However, some Dutch physicians may be too willing to ease death in response to a terminal care crisis that might be helped by the skilled, comprehensive application of palliative care. This could circumvent the human process of dying, depriving it of its mystery and its potential for healing and growth. If VAE and PAS are too readily available, the risk of subtle or explicit coercion of vulnerable patients increases. Easing death should never become too routinized, and the anguish physicians go through in conducting such an extraordinary act must never be played down. For this reason, some favor maintaining the criminal nature of the act, using the ensuing judicial follow-up as a safeguard. Whereas this ambiguous solution works reasonably well in the Netherlands, the legal system in the United States is more politicized and punitive and less predictable. Therefore, under similar legal circumstances, these practices would likely remain more secretive and idiosyncratic in the United States than in the Netherlands.

Responsiveness to Harsh Suffering at the End of Life

Most Dutch physicians enter into genuine partnerships with their patients, and they understand that part of their burden as physicians is to address unbearable suffering, even if it sometimes requires easing death. Many have an open mind about what kinds of suffering an individual patient might find intolerable, and are willing to give dying patients considerable leeway in determining when they have had enough. The notion that dying patients might have to take matters into their own hands because physicians are afraid to act is morally reprehensible to the Dutch. Similarly, giving a patient a lethal dose of medicine to take without being available to respond to problems would be considered both moral and professional malpractice.

In the United States, physicians are willing to go to extraordinary lengths to preserve and extend life. However, when a patient's personhood is disintegrating in the process of dying, our public policy and professional guidelines tend to be conservative and restrictive. Some patients in the United States are fortunate to have a long-term, committed relationship with their physician, but too often care is impersonal and episodic. Nevertheless, no matter how long or well a patient has been known in the past, if he or she is dying a bad death, it should be considered a medical emergency, requiring creative, flexible, continuous physician input until a solution is found.[72] If health care policy in the United States is not going to allow VAE or PAS as an escape of last resort when all other palliative measures fail, then guidelines about how doctors should respond must be developed. If answers in the United States to these devastating problems are to be TS and/or VSED, then whether they are morally different, less subject to abuse, and as acceptable to patients as VAE or PAS must be explored. Solutions must be made explicit with policies and safeguards, not only to protect patients against potential abuse but also to reassure the public that there can be a predictable escape under the worst imaginable circumstances. Patients in the United States must understand that physicians and policy makers are listening to and respecting their fears, and that the medical and legal professions will encourage responsiveness if suffering becomes unbearable. For most, reassurance will be all that is needed, because good palliative care is generally very effective. But dying patients need to know that there can be a humane, medically sanctioned escape if their suffering becomes intolerable in spite of the best palliative care possible. American physicians must demonstrate the same compassion and creative energy to relieve suffering that is currently shown in the fight for life.

References

1. de Wachter MAM. Active euthanasia in the Netherlands. *JAMA* 1989; 262:3316–3319.
2. Kimsma G, van Leeuwen E. Dutch euthanasia: Background, practice and present justifications. *Cambridge Quarterly of Healthcare Ethics* 1993; 2:19–35.
3. Battin MP. A dozen caveats concerning the discussion of euthanasia in the Netherlands. *Least Worst Death: Essays in Bioethics on the End of Life*. New York: Oxford University Press, 1994, pp. 130–144.
4. van der Wal G, Dillmann RJM. Euthanasia in the Netherlands. *Br Med J* 1994; 308:1346–1349.
5. Gomez C. Regulating Death: Euthanasia and the Case of the Netherlands. New York: Free Press, 1991.
6. Hendin H. Seduced by death: Doctors, patients and the Dutch cure. *Issues Law Med* 1994; 10:718–722.
7. Foley KM. Pain, physician-assisted suicide, and euthanasia. *Pain Forum* 1995; 4:163–178.
8. Gormally L. *Euthanasia, Clinical Practice and the Law*. London: The Linnacre Center, 1994.
9. Back AL, Wallace JI, Starks HE, Pearlman RA. Physician-assisted suicide and euthanasia in Washington State: Patient requests and physician responses. *JAMA* 1996; 275:919–925.
10. Meier DE, Emmons C, Wallenstein S, Quill TE, Morrison RS, Cassel CK. A national survey of physician-assisted suicide and euthanasia in the United States. *N Engl J Med* 1998; 338:1193–1201.
11. Chin AE, Hedberg K, Higginson GK, Fleming DW. Legalized physician-assisted suicide in Oregon—the first year's experience. *N Engl J Med* 1999; 340(7):577–583.
12. Sullivan AD, Hedberg K, Fleming DW. Legalized physician-assisted suicide in Oregon—The second year. *N Engl J Med* 2000; 342:598–604.
13. Jecker NS. Physician-assisted death in the Netherlands and the United States: Ethical and cultural aspects of policy development. *J Am Geriatr Soc* 1994; 42: 672–678.
14. Battin MP. The way we do it, the way they do it. *J Pain Symptom Manage* 1991; 6:298–305.
15. Fenigsen R. The Netherlands: new regulations concerning euthanasia. *Issues Law Med* 1993; 9:167–173.
16. van der Maas PJ, van Delden JJM, Pijnenborg L. *Euthanasia and Other Medical Decisions Concerning the End of Life: An Investigation*. New York: Elsevier, 1992.
17. van der Maas PJ, van der Wal G, Haverkate I, de Graaff CL, Kester JG, Onwuteaka-Philipsen BD, et al. Euthanasia, physician-assisted suicide, and other medical practices involving the end of life in the Netherlands, 1990–1995. *N Engl J Med* 1996; 335:1699–1705.
18. Kimsma G, Van Duin B. Teaching euthanasia. *Cambridge Quarterly of Healthcare Ethics* 1996; 5:107–113.
19. Quill TE, Cassel CK, Meier DE. Care of the hopelessly ill. Proposed criteria for physician-assisted suicide. *N Engl J Med* 1992; 327:1380–1384.
20. Miller FG, Quill TE, Brody H, Fletcher JC, Gostin LO, Meier DE. Regulating physician-assisted death. *N Engl J Med* 1994; 331:119–123.
21. Brody H. Assisted death: A compassionate response to a medical failure. *N Engl J Med* 1992; 327:1384–1385.

22. The SUPPORT Principal Investigators. A controlled trial to improve care for seriously ill hospitalized patients. The study to understand prognoses and preferences for outcomes and risks of treatment (SUPPORT). *JAMA* 1995; 274:1591–1598.

23. Dalen JE. US manpower needs. Generalists and specialists: achieving the balance. *Arch Intern Med* 1996; 156:21–24.

24. Billings JA, Block SD. Palliative care in undergraduate education: status report and future directions. *JAMA* 1997; 278:733–738.

25. Billings JA. Medical education for hospice care: A selected bibliography with brief annotations. *Hospice J* 1993; 9:69–83.

26. Dougherty C. Ethical values in health care reform. *JAMA* 1992; 268:2409–2412.

27. Rhymes J. Hospice care in America. *JAMA* 1990; 264:369–372.

28. Stoddard S. Hospice in the United States: An overview. *J Palliat Care* 1989; 5:10.

29. Christakis NA. Timing of referral of terminally ill patients to an outpatient hospice. *J Gen Intern Med* 1994; 9:314–320.

30. Lynn J. Caring at the end of our lives. *N Engl J Med* 1996; 335:201–202.

31. National Hospice Organization. (1990). Statement of the National Hospice Organization Opposing the Legalization of Euthanasia and Assisted Suicide.

32. Alpers A, Lo B. Physician-assisted suicide in Oregon: A bold experiment. *JAMA* 1995; 274:483–487.

33. *Vacco v. Quill*. 1997. 117 S.Ct. 2293.

34. *Washington v. Glucksberg*. 1997. 117 S.Ct. 2258.

35. Quill TE. Death and dignity: A case of individualized decision making. *N Engl J Med* 1991; 324:691–694.

36. Gostin LO. Life and death choices after Cruzan. *Law Med Health Care* 1991; 19:9–12.

37. Newman S. Euthanasia: Orchestrating "the last syllable of . . . time." *University Pittsburgh Law Rev* 1991; 53:153–191.

38. Hemlock Society. *1991 Roper Poll of the West Coast on Euthanasia*. New York: Roper Organization, 1991.

39. Blendon RJ, Szalay US, Knox RA. Should physicians aid their patients in dying? The public perspective. *JAMA* 1992; 267:2658–2662.

40. Blackhall LJ, Murphy ST, Frank G, Michel V, Azan S. Ethnicity and attitudes toward patient autonomy. *JAMA* 1995; 274:820–825.

41. Cohen JS, Fihn SD, Boyko EJ, Jonsen AR, Wood RW. Attitudes toward assisted suicide and euthanasia among physicains in Washington State. *N Engl J Med* 1994; 331:89–94.

42. Lukes S. *Individualism*. Oxford: Blackwell, 1973.

43. Schneewind JB. The use of autonomy in ethical theory. In: Heller TC, Sosna M, Wellberry DE, editors. *Reconstructing Individualism: Autonomy, Individualism, and the Self in Western Thought*. Stanford, Calif.: Stanford University Press, 1986.

44. Beauchamp TL, Childress JF. *Principles of Biomedical Ethics*. New York: Oxford University Press, 1994.

45. Hooykaas R. *Religion and the Rise of Modern Science*. Edinburg and London: Scottish Academy Press, 1972.

46. Gottleib BR. Abortion—1995. *N Engl J Med* 1995; 332:532–533.

47. Quill TE, Dresser R, Brock DW. Rule of double effect: A critique of its role in end-of-life decision making. *N Engl J Med* 1997; 337:1768–1771.

48. Quill TE. Principle of double effect and end-of-life pain management: Additional myths and a limited role. *J Palliat Med* 1998; 2:333–336.

49. Marquis DB. Four versions of the double effect. *J Med Philos* 1991; 16:515–544.
50. Brody H. Causing, intending and assisting death. *J Clin Ethics* 1993; 4:112–117.
51. Quill TE. The ambiguity of clinical intentions. *N Engl J Med* 1993; 329:1039–1040.
52. Gevers JKM. Legislation on euthanasia: Recent developments in the Netherlands. *J Med Ethics* 1992; 18:138–141.
53. Welie JVM. The medical exception: Physicians, euthanasia and the Dutch criminal law. *J Med Philos* 1992; 17:419–437.
54. Leenen HJJ. *Handboek gezondheidsrecht (Handbook on Healthlaw)*. Samson: Alphen aan de Rhijn, 1988.
55. Hendin H, Rutenfrans C, Zylicz Z. Physician-assisted suicide and euthanasia in the Netherlands. Lessons from the Dutch. *JAMA* 1997; 277:1720–1722.
56. Neu S, Kjellstrand CM. Stopping long-term dialysis. Am empirical study of withdrawal of life-supporting treatment. *N Engl J Med* 1986; 314:14–20.
57. Cohen LM, McCue JD, Germain M, Kjellstrand CM. Dialysis discontinuation. A "good" death? *Arch Intern Med* 1995; 155:42–47.
58. Prendergast TJ, Luce JM. Increasing incidence of withholding and withdrawal of life support from the critically ill. *Am J Respir Crit Care Med* 1997; 115:15–20.
59. Quill TE, Byock I. Responding to intractable terminal suffering: The role of terminal sedation and voluntary refusal of food and fluids. ACP-ASIM End-of-Life Care Consensus Panel. *Ann Intern Med* 2000; 132:408–414.
60. Ventafridda V, Ripamonti C, DeConno F, Tamburini M, Cassileth BR. Symptom prevalence and control during cancer patients' last days of life. *J Palliat Care* 1990; 6:7–11.
61. Troug RD, Berde DB, Mitchell C, Grier HE. Barbiturates in the care of the terminally ill. *N Engl J Med* 1991; 327:1678–1682.
62. Lee MA, Tolle SW. Oregon's assisted suicide vote: The silver lining. *Ann Intern Med* 1996; 124:267–269.
63. Tolle SW, Rosenfeld AG, Tilden VP, Park Y. Oregon's low in-hospital death rates: What determines where people die and satisfaction with decisions on place of death? *Ann Intern Med* 1999; 130:681–685.
64. Billings JA, Block SD. Slow euthanasia. *J Palliat Care* 1996; 12:21–30.
65. Quill TE. *Death and Dignity: Making Choices and Taking Charge*. New York: W.W. Norton and Co., 1993.
66. Buchanan A, Brock D. *Deciding for Others: The Ethics of Surrogate Decision Making*. Cambridge: Cambridge University Press, 1989.
67. Angell M. Euthanasia in the Netherlands—good news or bad? *N Engl J Med* 1996; 335:1676–1678.
68. Jochemsen H. Euthanasia in Holland: an ethical critique of the new law. *J Med Ethics* 1994; 20:212–217.
69. Klotzko AJ, Chabot B. Arlene Judith Klotzko and Dr. Boudewijn Chabot discuss assisted suicide in the absence of somatic illness. *Cambridge Quarterly of Healthcare Ethics* 1995; 4:239–249.
70. Quill TE, Cassel CK. Nonabandonment: A central obligation for physicians. *Ann Intern Med* 1995; 122:368–374.
71. Meisel A, Snyder L, Quill TE. Seven legal barriers to end-of-life care: Myths, realities, and grains of truth. *JAMA* 2000; 284:2495–2501.
72. Quill TE, Brody RV. "You promised me I wouldn't die like this." A bad death as a medical emergency. *Arch Intern Med* 1995; 155:1250–1254.

Epilogue

All About My Brother

It started with a phone call in the middle of the night. *"Don has been in a biking accident. He was hit by a car and has broken a lot of bones and badly injured his head. I'm heading to the hospital."* Oh my God! How quickly one's life can change! I get phone calls in the middle of the night about other people's tragedies, but I have never been on the receiving end of devastating news that hit so close to home.

Toni, my brother's wife, gave me the phone number of the Surgical Intensive Care Unit at Massachusetts General Hospital, where Don had been airlifted. I spoke with one of the nurses. *"It doesn't look too good. His pupils were fixed and dilated when he came in, and he has blood around and inside of his brain. He is unconscious, and the neurosurgeons and trauma team are evaluating him."* Fixed and dilated! Sometimes it may be better not to have too much medical knowledge. The pupillary light reflexes of the eyes are among the most primitive in the brain, and they are compromised only with the severest of brain injuries.

This news was so overwhelming that it was hard to decide how to proceed. My heart was racing and I was shaking as I called my other brother, Steve, in Arizona. We decided to call my parents together that night rather than wait until we arrived in Boston the next morning. It was possible that Don would not survive the night, and they needed to know—in spite of how painful it would be. A parent's worst nightmare began with that call. Our parents headed to the hospital, and our most trying adventure ever as a family was under way.

I had planned a trip to Philadelphia for the next day to participate in a round-table discussion, "Fred Friendly" style, about end-of-life care. This is not my favorite forum, because there is a tendency for participants to debate in terms of sharp, clever one-liners that can easily overshadow the core issues at stake. Through a quick turn of fate, I was going to be living critical end-of-life decision making around a person whom I loved dearly, and whose fate would lie in the balance. I wished I could go back to sleep and wake up in a different time and place. Perhaps this was just a bad dream.

Who was my brother Don, and how did he arrive at this moment?

Don was the youngest of three children, all boys. As the youngest sibling by more than seven years, Don missed much of the competitive horseplay that his oldest brother, Steve, and I indulged in. Don was very independent as a child, and tended to keep his thoughts and feelings to himself. He quietly avoided being the center of attention, and was usually surrounded by a small group of good friends.

Our father's position with General Electric required transfers to different cities about every three years. Our travels eventually took us to the North Shore of Boston when Don was nine years old. He took to sailing immediately, and would spend as much time on the water, in sailboats of all sizes and makes, as my parents would allow. Even in heavy winds, Don was as comfortable sailing in a crowded harbor as he was on the high seas. While in college, Don took a year off from school to skipper large boats down the East Coast to the Caribbean.

When Don found something he liked, he did it full bore. He would fully prepare himself with knowledge and proper equipment, then progressively develop his proficiency. He loved the latest and best equipment, and would use it to its full potential. Don eventually took up windsurfing, and he progressed in characteristic fashion to tiny boards, light sails, and high winds. Don would windsurf in the ocean anytime the winds were high enough, in summer or winter. Several times he headed to the Columbia River Gorge for a quick "vaca-tion"; there he would windsurf in the heavy winds from dawn to dusk for days on end.

Don and Toni met at the beginning of law school. Toni had a love of the envi-ronment and nature, and eventually went to work for the Environmental Pro-tection Agency. Don was never able to merge his vocation with his avocations. As a corporate lawyer, Don worked on many major commercial real estate transactions around Boston and the Northeast, but his main passions remained with the sea. Don would sometimes leave work in the middle of the day when the winds were high enough to go windsurfing, and later return to the office and work until the middle of the night to more than make up for the lost time.

Don and Toni made trips all over the world—the necessary ingredients being consistently high winds and untarnished natural habitats.

As a young man, Don had difficulty recognizing his own needs and wants. As he grew older, he gradually learned to identify and then follow his own interests. He became adamant about protecting time to explore his passions, and Toni fortunately gave him the space to be himself in this regard. After being together for more than 15 years, Don and Toni eventually "eloped" and later had a party to allow family and friends to celebrate the evolution of their relationship. Don remained quiet in a crowd, and didn't like being the center of attention. But with his close friends, he was open and articulate. And on a windsurfer or in a boat, his actions were anything but reserved.

Eight months before Don's accident, with Toni's biological clock rapidly ticking, Toni and Don gave birth to their first child, David John. Our parents had already sold their house in Connecticut and moved back to the North Shore, only a few miles from Don and Toni. The move turned out to be better than expected on all accounts, and Dave's birth shortly thereafter seemed to be the crowning event. Our parents were totally and unequivocally in love with Dave—we had never seen them happier. Pictures of Don and Dave as infants were indistinguishable, and Toni had presented baby pictures of Don and Dave side by side to our parents as gifts. Don became very connected to Dave, and seemed more content than I had seen him in years. His plate was very full with parenting, work, and his various avocations, but Don had no shortage of energy.

About eight years ago, Don took up mountain biking. He went at this sport with his usual zeal, quickly becoming proficient and challenging himself with progressively steeper hills and more rugged terrain. In characteristic fashion, he became a student of the sport, obtained the latest in high-tech equipment, and utilized it to its potential. In recent years, Don turned his attention to long-distance bicycle touring. He and his riding friends would think nothing of riding 40 to 50 miles per day on the weekend. They would make an annual ride from Boston to Provincetown, and return by ferryboat the same day. The physical challenge, beautiful landscape, and combination of biking and boating made this a peak experience for Don.

On the night of the accident, Don got home a little earlier than usual. He told Toni he wanted to take a bike ride. He spent some time with Dave, took care of some chores, put his bike in his truck, and eventually headed off to a nearby area where there are some excellent country roads for riding. It was a beautiful, warm evening, and the sun was just beginning to set. I would like to think he felt on top of the world. Don had only been riding for 10 to 15 minutes when he came down a gentle hill into a seemingly innocent crossroads. The trees were just starting to bud, and spring was in the air. There was a beautiful meadow to the left, and trees obscured the view farther down the road.

The next moment transformed the lives of our family forever. A confluence of unfortunate forces and circumstances merged at that dangerous intersection. Don was coming down the hill on a road that dead-ended at the intersection. An 18 year-old boy was driving much too fast down the intersecting country road, followed closely by friends in a second car. Within seconds, there was a broken windshield and a shattered bicycle helmet, and Don was lying facedown in a water-filled ditch on the opposite side of the road. Long skid marks caused by locked brakes could be seen on the left side of the road, then swerving farther left.

Within 30 minutes, a helicopter arrived to transport Don directly to the Surgical Intensive Care Unit at Massachusetts General Hospital. Such high-tech centers are where you would hope a loved one involved in such a serious accident would receive care. Don was admitted to the hospital as a "John Doe" because he was found with no identifying data.

Toni had put Dave to bed then had gone to bed herself, tired from a long day of work and parenting. She awoke later that evening, became frightened because she could not find Don, and decided to call the police. Shortly thereafter, the local police came to her house and informed her of Don's accident and his admission to Massachusetts General Hospital.

We headed to the hospital from different parts of the country, hoping for the best but preparing for the worst. The words "fixed and dilated" clattered in my brain as I tried to prepare myself for what we would find. Perhaps these ominous reflexes were a result of acute brain swelling that might be reversible. If not, Don was in real trouble.

When my wife, Penny, and I arrived, the waiting room was filled. Toni, my mother and aunt, and several of Toni and Don's closest friends were there. Everyone was exhausted, apprehensive, and somewhat dazed. It had been the longest of nights. *"Don doesn't look very good—all swollen, banged up, and not responsive."* We had to ask permission from the medical staff to see Don, and were informed that he would not be "ready to be seen" for 20 to 30 minutes. They would call us in the waiting room when they had him ready. As we were each trying to hold our emotions in check for one another's benefit, waves of anxiety, sadness, and fear emerged. At the slightest provocation, one of us would break down, to be comforted by another. This kind of emotional rawness was somewhat unfamiliar to our rather stoical family, yet there was no way (and no reason) to hide the grief that was all around us.

I tried to steel myself as I approached Don's room. In my work as a physician, I have seen severe trauma and been able to isolate myself from my own feelings to do what had to be done. However, this was my kid brother, and there was no way to shield myself from the enormity of the loss.

Don was almost unrecognizable. His left leg was casted, he had chest tubes in both lungs, and he was on a mechanical ventilator. His face, neck, and upper body were extremely swollen, and he had a large bruise on the left side of his head. A decompressing "bolt" had been put directly into the top of his head in an attempt to relieve the pressure buildup caused by the trauma and bleeding in his brain. Other than a slight involuntary twitch when we touched his right hand, Don was incredibly still.

Don's primary nurse was constantly at his bedside, attending to the multiple monitors, medical lines, and medication drips. She explained to us what was being attempted medically, and expressed her condolences. At first, the shock of seeing Don made our brains unreceptive to any information. Eventually I asked, *"Is he responding at all?"* The nurse said we could talk to the neuro-surgeon later in the day when he finished the morning's surgery, but so far he had exhibited only a few spontaneous breaths, and maybe a gag reflex. *"What about his eyes?"* I asked. *"Are they still fixed and dilated?"* The nurse responded that they had not been checked since early in the night because of the facial swelling, but as far as she knew there were no changes. *Oh my God!* My brain was ringing out and numb at the same time. I felt like screaming, but found myself mute. I wanted to say something encouraging to Don but couldn't find the words. I simply whispered to him that I loved him, and I started to cry. I found an uninjured spot to kiss above his right eyebrow, then left his side to face the other members of our family.

Although I was determined to be a brother and not a doctor to Don, it was impossible to put my medical expertise completely away. I would be the trans-lator for our family about the meaning and extent of Don's injuries. Clearly understanding Don's medical condition and prognosis would be critical to making sense of what had happened, and eventually to make decisions on his behalf. I did not mind taking on this role that I knew so well from my professional work. It allowed me to help care for Don when there seemed so little else I could do. Nevertheless, I definitely did not want to be the sole family decision maker for Don, and I hoped we could work together to achieve a consensus of opinion about how Don would want us to proceed.

"What do you think?" our family and friends assembled in the waiting room asked when Penny and I returned from Don's bedside. They knew my answer by looking at my face, but hearing it is another matter. I needed to tell them the truth without bludgeoning them with it. *"He doesn't appear to be suffer-ing, but it doesn't look good at all. Don is in real trouble. He is in the best of hands, and they are doing all they can. His head injury is very severe; the rest of his body could probably survive, but his brain has been badly damaged."* Fortunately I was not telling our family members anything they did not already know, yet because of my medical background, hearing my perceptions was deflating for them. My mother confided that she felt he was "already gone" when she saw him. My experience in end-of-life care made me apprehensive about the daunting decisions we would have to face over the next hours or days, but I promised myself to take it moment by moment rather than look too far down the road.

The surgical intensive care unit had a unique culture. The nursing staff was its heart and soul. The primary nurses were extremely technically competent, and they were given a lot of responsibility in managing the medical details of Don's care. They were also very respectful of Don as a human being and of us as a family. They would ask how we were doing, try to respond to our questions, and give us guidance about what to expect next. The identity of the primary nurse was never in doubt; at change of shift, one primary nurse would say good-bye and introduce us to the next one. The commitments of partnership and nonabandonment were clearly fulfilled with this part of the staff.

The physicians were also excellent technically. Biomedical expertise was especially critical at this early juncture. We needed to be sure that everything possible was being done medically to sustain Don, and to allow his brain to recover if that was possible. Don had multiple teams of physicians, including experts in trauma, ICU, neurosurgery, neurology, and orthopedics, overseeing the separate aspects of his care. Each team had interns, residents, fellows, and a senior physician, but no one was identified as Don's main doctor or as a coordinator among the specialists. It was not clear who, if anyone, among the physicians was empowered to make decisions with us, or to discuss Don's overall clinical condition and prognosis. This could be very dangerous for Don, but we decided to take a wait-and-see approach—in part because we were all too much in shock to try to take charge.

There were moments of humanity and caring among the medical and nursing staffs that made a huge difference. A young ICU physician whom I helped train in Rochester was one of the doctors who had worked on Don when he first came in. He approached us and said, *"I am so sorry. I wish we could do more. It is so frustrating to not be able to help such a young, active person when we frequently spend so much time treating those whose potential seems so much less."* Others offered informal conversation, condolences about our loss, food and drink, a comfortable chair, or a warm blanket. These small touches helped to humanize a process that otherwise seemed so cruel and unfair.

Critical Moments in Decision Making

Don was clearly not in a position to make decisions for himself in the hospital. As his family, we therefore had to decide how Don would want to proceed if he could understand his condition and speak for himself. Initially we were not sure if Don had completed a living will, or if he had named anyone to be his health care proxy, but we all knew that Don valued his physical and mental integrity, and that he would not want to be kept alive indefinitely in a vegetative state. Beyond that, we knew little about the specifics of his wishes in this particular circumstance. Yet decisions would have to be made. We would have to achieve a consensus about how to proceed, guided by our perceptions of Don's values and wishes, as well as a clear understanding of his clinical condition and prognosis.

What follows are a few of the critical issues that we had to consider on Don's behalf:

1. *The full-court press*: From the outset, Don received any and all medical interventions that might help him to survive. He was put on a breathing machine, and tubes were inserted into his chest to expand his collapsed lungs. He had a "bolt" drain and monitor placed directly into his brain in an attempt to reduce his elevated intracranial pressure. Multiple lines were introduced into his veins to deliver medications to maintain the circulation to his brain while reducing its pressure. Neurosurgeons contemplated surgically draining the blood from around his brain, while orthopedists placed a temporary cast on his leg. As long as there was a chance of recovery, this invasion of Don's body had meaning and was appropriate. As long as the goal was an all-out fight to preserve Don's life, his consent to these invasive procedures was assumed. Fortunately, Don did not appear to be suffering. Yet terrible questions lurked just under the surface. *How badly was his brain injured? How likely was his recovery? What might recovery mean? What if his body recovered but his brain did not? What if his brain only partially recovered and he was left alive but unable to move, think, or interact?* And on and on. . . . Although we vowed to take it one step at a time, we would soon have to address some of these questions to properly advocate for Don.

2. *What was Don's prognosis?* Don had been in the Surgical Intensive Care Unit for about 12 hours when I arrived. He had minimal, if any, basic brain stem reflexes, and no sign of higher cortical function. We would have to wait for the senior neurosurgeon to answer further questions. The neurosurgical resident eventually came to speak with us, and he confirmed the worst. Don's pupils were still "fixed and dilated," and his eyes had no response when his corneas were touched. He still would gag a little when his throat was stimulated, and he had a small amount of spontaneous breathing. I asked Toni if I could ask the resident some hard questions. When she nodded, I steeled myself to give voice to the questions and to listen carefully to the answers. *"Is there any sign of higher brain function?" "No." "Is there any significant chance of recovering higher brain functioning?" "Unfortunately, I don't think so. His brain has been severely injured in his dominant hemisphere. I can show you the scan if*

*it would be helpful." "What would be the best we could hope for in terms
of brain function?" "I would have to wait for my supervisor to give you
a final answer on that, but it would probably be some variation of a persistent vegetative state."* At this point we had heard enough. This information was hard to accept, but it was important that it be delivered as
clearly and unequivocally as possible. I was very grateful to this resident
for being honest with us, and for having the courage to answer our
questions directly. We now knew what we were facing, which would help
determine the next steps we would take. I asked the resident if this was
the kind of situation in which organ donation could be considered. He
responded in the affirmative.

3. *The core decision makers*: A private meeting of the immediate family was
necessary so we could discuss what we had learned. I was familiar with
this process from my work as a clinician, but now it was my own family,
and my younger brother's well-being was at stake. Don's doctors had
been called away, so I would have to translate what had been said,
and help interpret what it meant. Toni was a central decision maker as
Don's wife, as were Steve and I as Don's brothers. Our goal was to seek
consensus among immediate family members at each step along the way.
Our parents, my wife Penny, and one of our aunts were also there to ask
questions, provide support, and witness the process. I reiterated what our
job was: to make decisions as Don would if he could understand his situation and speak for himself. We all agreed that Don would not want to
be kept alive if he had no chance of regaining consciousness and participating fully in life. If that was not possible, then we should stop aggressive treatment and keep him comfortable. Our family also agreed that
Don would want us to pursue organ donation if what we had learned about
his prognosis was true. We would await the final word from the senior
neurosurgeon, who would meet with us later in the day, and then make
our decision.

4. *A change in strategy*: It was late afternoon before we met with the
neurosurgeon. Toni had had enough medical conversation and preferred
to spend her time at Don's bedside. Steve, Penny, and I met with the
doctor, who started with generalities about Don "not looking too good"
and later gently confirmed what his resident had told us earlier in the
day. The best we could hope for would be some kind of persistent
vegetative state, but even that was improbable given Don's degree of
injury. At this point we asked that Don be evaluated for organ donation.
If that was not possible, we said, we wanted all life-sustaining therapy
stopped so that Don could be allowed to die peacefully. We asked
that the transplant team be called immediately, as we did not want Don
to suffer unnecessarily and we did not want the opportunity to donate

his organs to be lost. We learned that Don would have to lose his few remaining brain stem reflexes to be a candidate for transplant. This would take an undetermined period of time—perhaps hours or days. The goal of treatment would now shift toward preserving his other organs rather than his brain, and his medications and medical support systems would be adjusted accordingly. Steve and I informed the rest of the family and Don's friends about what we had learned. Everyone was sad, but no one was particularly surprised.

5. *The transplant team takes over*: Early in Don's course of treatment, there were many doctors but no chief decision makers. Now the transplant coordinators were a continuous presence for our family for the remainder of Don's time in the hospital. They were very helpful in telling us what the steps were, and arranging for us to spend as much time with Don as possible. We learned that the absence of brain function would have to be confirmed by a senior neurologist before transplant could occur, but that they could begin the blood typing and testing for infection. As soon as brain function ceased, they would begin the search for suitably matched organ recipients and do some final tests of organ function. Don seemed to be stabilizing from a cardiovascular point of view, so we would now begin waiting with a mind-set not of his recovery but of his imminent death. We split responsibilities so that everyone would have some support and get some rest. Steve would stay with our parents, who were mentally and physically exhausted. Toni and Penny would stay with the baby. Don and Toni's friends—Bill, Mary Ellen, and Chris—would be on call in case we needed to act in the middle of the night. I would stay with Don. Today had been the longest and most difficult day in all of our lives, and tomorrow would likely be no different.

6. *Preparing for death*: Don's blood pressure became unstable during the middle of the night. The senior neurologist was called in, and he confirmed that Don had lost his remaining brain stem reflexes. Don was now officially "brain dead," so the process of organ donation could formally move forward. Don's blood pressure and heart rate eventually stabilized, so we could wait until morning. The staff set up a Geri-chair so I could spend the night at Don's side. This was of immeasurable help in my coming to grips with Don's impending death. The nursing staff was kind and accommodating, watching over Don's medical condition while taking me under their wing with supportive comments, warm blankets, and coffee. In the early morning, Don passed (or failed) the final test of brain death by not breathing for six minutes when taken off his mechanical ventilator. The final phase of preparation for organ donation was soon under way: function tests of his injured lungs, as well as of his heart, liver, pancreas, and kidneys.

Toni, Steve, Penny, Bill, Chris, and I spent most of the next day sitting with Don. The anxiety we had each felt upon first seeing Don injured, and attached to so much technology, began to fade. We began to reminisce, tell stories about Don and ourselves, laugh, and cry. Thankfully, multiple delays in the preparation process allowed us to spend extra hours with Don. Whereas the preceding day had been interminable, this day went by quickly. At times, we tried to imagine the excitement of the people who were being notified that a long-awaited, potentially lifesaving organ would soon be available. How strange life is that our tragedy could result in their salvation!

7. *Time to say good-bye*: Saying good-bye to Don was the saddest thing I have ever done. A final test (a portable CT scan of his lungs) kept being postponed, giving us extra time with him. Yet eventually the moment arrived. The testing had been completed, and the transplant surgeons were waiting. We found ourselves quietly crying at different times during the day, sometimes triggered by a most inconsequential thought or statement. We would hug or touch one another, then move on. As we began our final good-byes, our sobs were unrestrained. *Good luck. I hope the wind is howling. I love you. You are a great person. I will miss you. We will watch over Dave for you.* We kissed Don good-bye, we hugged one another and many of the staff who had been so helpful, and then we stumbled out of the hospital into the brilliant sunlight. It was the most intense and heartbreaking experience any of us had ever been through. A lot of our own hearts and souls were left behind.

Unfinished Business

When someone dies suddenly, there are always regrets. Sudden death may be easier on the person who dies than a more prolonged death, but it is rarely easier on the family. I wish I had told Don more explicitly that I loved and respected him. I wish I had attended Don and Toni's wedding celebration instead of being too busy with my own life. I had recently bought an espresso machine at Don's recommendation that I was enjoying thoroughly, and I had thought of calling him to say thanks, but I never did. Each of us who loved Don has gone through a similar process. We were completely unprepared for his death, and had missed opportunities to let him know how much we cared about him.

Keeping Don's spirit alive for Dave is now a major commitment. I had not known Toni too well before the accident, but I now know her much better, and am connected to her and Dave for life. The "Don Stories" from his friends and colleagues will be formally collected as a way of keeping his memory vivid for

Dave. Don's legend will reach mythic proportions if we have anything to do with it. I had previously thought a lot about what it means to be a good father to my two daughters. Penny and I now think much more carefully about what it means to be present as aunt and uncle to Dave than we otherwise would have. Steve's and my responsibility to our parents and to each other has also grown more complex with Don's absence. There is something unnatural about losing a child, even when that child is 43, and our parents will need all the love and support they can find from family and friends to survive this loss.

Can we find forgiveness for the 18 year-old boy who was driving much too fast on that country road? He apparently was not drunk or on drugs. We do not know his state of mind, but there was probably no malicious intent. Speeding and cutting curves on a narrow country road were very stupid things to do, but many of us have been on similar roads under similar circumstances, and had near misses. I would not want to be in his shoes, and have to make peace with his role in this tragedy; I can even feel some sadness for him. I also understand that the forces that brought Don to that crossroads were much bigger than his actions alone.

Finally, and perhaps most challengingly, I felt a brief surge of anger toward Don when I first learned of his accident. How could he have risked so much with his fervor for bicycle touring when he had so much to lose? Yet everything I have subsequently learned about Don from his fellow riders and windsurfers suggests that he was not reckless. The edges he was testing were of his own endurance and skill. He did not like to bike in traffic, and he enjoyed the physical challenge of a long hill climb much more that the thrill of speeding downhill. He took terrific care of his body and his equipment, and he loved discovering their potentials. Don lived life fully. He was a model for all of us with respect to identifying one's passions, then exploring them with enthusiasm and skill.

Where Do We Find Hope?

If I had faith in an all-powerful, beneficent God, that faith would have been shaken to the core with Don's accident. I do not think She would allow such things to happen. I know that bad things happen to good people, and that life can sometimes be perverse and unfair. Certainly life can be mercurial and fragile. Don approached life with intensity and passion. Think how much more tragic his death would have been if he did not leave work in the middle of the day when the wind was roaring, or if he had been saving his best for a retirement that never came. Don led a good and full life, caring for himself as well as others, following many of his dreams. His death was a tragic loss for all of us, but he made the most of the time he had.

Our family was severely tested in this tragedy, and came through with flying colors. Toni showed a courage and depth of thought and feeling at which I can only marvel. She was an inspiration to us all as she painfully came to grips with the loss of her lover and friend, then helped to make the decision to set him free and allow others to have the gift of his organs. My parents often commented on how lucky we had been as a family to have avoided such losses in the past. They found a way to keep going in spite of the enormity of their grief, and to make some sense of Don's death despite the fact that it does not make sense. They need only look at Dave to have a reason to go on. My brother Steve was also present emotionally and physically throughout the ordeal. Despite the fact that he had no medical background, he asked hard questions and tried to comprehend the meaning of the answers. My wife, Penny, was at my side throughout, providing support where it was needed, whether it was to my parents, Toni, Dave, Steve, or me. Finally, my children, Carrie and Megan, came as soon as possible, and added immeasurably to the atmosphere of support, sadness, and hope. Though it is sometimes easy to focus on family foibles, this experience made me proud to be a member of our clan, and more respectful and understanding of the importance of family.

Don's death also reinforced the importance of community. Don and Toni's wonderful friends were at Toni's side throughout those awful two days, and in the bereavement period thereafter. Bill and Chris stayed with us at Don's bedside for his last day, and helped Toni remember that others cared about both her and Don. Bill's wife, Mary Ellen, took care of Dave so that Toni could feel assured he was in the best of hands. Their other friends were present in the background, available at a moment's notice to help in any way they could. My aunt Anna was at my mother's side, making sure that she always had a shoulder to lean on. Reverend Mary Harrington and other members of my parents' Unitarian Church were readily available with food and support, and helped to arrange a very personalized, moving memorial service. Finally, our friends back in Rochester were ready to assist from afar, and continued to support us once we returned home. This kind of tragedy brings out the best in people and makes you realize the importance of connection to local communities.

Of course, our greatest sources of hope are probably the laugh and smile of Don and Toni's son, Dave. In the grieving process, there are waves of anguish and despair that emerge out of the blue. We would sometimes be mired in sadness and loss when Dave was brought into the room; his bright eyes and joyous smile would help us emerge, at least temporarily, from our grief. The virtually identical pictures of Don and David as infants sitting in my parents' living room make even the non-Buddhists among us wonder about reincarnation, and certainly help to remind us that Don's spirit will live on in his son. Although Dave's existence makes Don's loss in many ways harder and more tragic, his presence reminds us that Don's life force will go on. Our job now is to help Dave grow up to be the best person he can be. We will let him know what a wonderful person his dad was, and how much he loved his young son.

Some of the hope we found was in the dark corners of the experience, and are not readily obvious to those who have not been through similar experiences. Beyond the split second of the accident, Don probably had no conscious awareness of what happened. He did not appear to suffer despite his catastrophic injuries and all of the invasive treatment that he required. He was cared for at Massachusetts General Hospital, a medical mecca for trauma, so there was no doubt that he received the best of care. The staff at the surgical intensive care unit, particularly the nurses, was technically very skilled, but also very respectful to Don and to us as his family. We were lucky in a way that Don's prognosis was clear, for it allowed us to proceed with decision making that included the opportunity to donate his organs. Some of the terrible "what ifs" in this scenario (*What if his brain stem continued to function without higher brain activity?* and *What if he had a little movement but was unable to think or communicate?*) never came to pass. Under those circumstances, our decision making would have been even more daunting, both existentially and morally. Finally, we found meaning in the opportunity to donate his organs. Sitting at Don's bedside, we allowed ourselves to imagine at least some of the excitement that the recipients had to be feeling at the same time we were preparing to let him go. Don was so physically fit and full of life at the time of his death that we all remarked about the extraordinary good fortune of the person who received his heart.

I learned from Don something about life's frailty and unpredictability, but also about living life to the fullest, and listening to one's own heart and instincts. Don began to understand himself relatively late in life, and once he did, he started to follow his own path more clearly. The road was bumpy at first, and dominated by an intensification of his athletic interests. But listening more carefully to his heart led to his marriage to Toni and eventually to Dave's birth. In his last years, Don was happier and more fulfilled than I had ever seen him. It seems a shame that he was taken at such a prime time in his life, but my guess is that he would have few regrets about his last years.

Reconciliation of Don's Death and My Beliefs about End-of-Life Care

Don's untimely death and the decision making that we faced as a family provide a reality check for the ideas presented in this book. Don died as I was about to compose this final chapter. The preceding chapters were already complete.

Since my life so radically changed as a result of his death, it seemed only fitting to close with an exploration of this experience. Let me end this chapter with some final reflections about each section of the book from the perspective of what we learned as a family from Don's death and his medical care.

Humanistic care starts with technical competence. We needed to know that everything possible was being done to medically support Don and help him recover. When he was not improving, there was no doubt the cause was his head injuries and not inadequate medical care. Once we understood that he was not going to recover in a way that would allow for a meaningful life, we then had to enter the complex ethical and legal arena of stopping treatment for a patient who cannot speak for himself. Again, because his clinical situation was clear, his options were quite limited: (1) continue aggressive care despite the fact that his brain would not recover, (2) stop aggressive care and withdraw life-sustaining therapy, or (3) explore organ donation. None of these options was particularly appealing, but it was evident to us as a family that organ donation was by far the best of the choices available.

Once technical and ethical competence was assured, the humanness with which we were treated made a major difference. In the early going, as we were trying to integrate and understand what had happened, the primary nurses in the surgical intensive care were invaluable. There was no doubt that they were in charge at the bedside, and that they were committed to caring for Don. They also treated Don and the rest of the family with kindness and respect. They let us know what to expect next, and answered our questions with honesty and caring. At the change of shift, they would introduce us to the next person who would be caring for Don. In terms of partnership, commitment, and nonabandonment, they were exemplary.

The many physicians involved in Don's care were also very technically competent. Unfortunately, there was never a single medical person identified who would be the ultimate arbiter of his care, both with us as his family and with the multiple medical teams involved. One of the medical physicians in the intensive care unit who had worked on Don when he first came in went out of his way to make contact with me, expressing his sorrow and keeping us informed about Don's situation, as did one of the neurologists. These moments of kindness and humanity made a huge difference to me as a person, but they did not make up for the absence of a clearly identified, responsible physician who might have created a partnership with us as a family to try to make decisions on Don's behalf. Because the decisions were relatively clear-cut, and because I had a considerable amount of medical experience, this omission was not as dangerous as it might have been if we had to make decisions that were ambiguous medically, ethically, or personally. When the transplant team became involved, they clearly served these coordinating, communicating, and

caring functions. We knew whom to talk to if we had concerns, and we understood they would be present for us all the way through until Don's death. My
belief in the centrality of partnership and nonabandonment are undiminished
by this experience.

The communication issues described in Part II were pivotal during our
ordeal. If we were to make sound decisions on Don's behalf, we needed
accurate and honest information at the same time that we were reeling from
our loss. Bad news is always painful to hear, and it is important to deliver it at
a pace determined by the patient's clinical circumstances and by the patient's
and family's readiness. Once I heard "fixed and dilated" over the phone, I began
to understand the probable enormity of what had happened, and I contemplated this as I was making arrangements to fly to Boston. When I saw Don,
his appearance confirmed my worst fears, but I needed to again confirm what
I thought was happening. The first pass at information was general and ambiguous *("It doesn't look too good. He has been severely injured.")*. Although I
personally needed to hear more specifics, I checked with Toni and Penny about
the advisability, as they saw it, of asking harder questions. When they both
nodded "okay," I asked more specifically about Don's higher brain function and
other brain stem reflexes, and I heard the truth about the extent of Don's
injuries and just how bad his prognosis was. The resident we were talking
with did an excellent job of allowing us to determine the pace of our discussion and the depth of the information we received, while remaining honest
and direct in response to our questions. Had we not had the medical experience to ask hard questions, and had we not been realistic about what we
were hearing, the pace at which we received this information might have been
overwhelming. However, any attempt by the doctors to keep the information ambiguous to protect us from the truth we needed to hear would have
infuriated us. Armed with accurate information, as a family we could begin to
address the reality and extent of our loss, and prepare to face the next stages
of decision making.

Because Don could not speak for himself, we had to represent him as best
we could. Toni did not think he had an advance directive, though we later
learned that he did. Therefore, we adopted a consensus approach among
immediate family who knew Don best, applying the principle of substituted
judgment. Even had we known of his advance directive, we would have used
the same approach, since the advance directive did not specifically address his
particular circumstance and the choices we faced. Once we fully understood
his prognosis for recovery of higher brain function, it was clear to all of us that
Don would not want to be kept alive in such a condition. If his prognosis
was clear, then the decision was simple, at least intellectually. The sadness
attached to such a decision is deep and unnerving, yet we had all worked hard
to understand what had happened, had supported each other, and had built

consensus about how to proceed. The expressions of sorrow and loss made by many of the nurses and physicians helped to reassure us that we were in this trying situation with humane professionals.

We were then faced with clinical and ethical dilemmas similar to those presented in Part III. Finding the least harmful way to help Don die in a way that would preserve his dignity and enhance the meaning of his life was our challenge. Once his brain stem function was completely gone, our choices were limited to discontinuing life-sustaining therapy, which would surely end in his death (he had already "failed" the apnea test), or keeping him alive with intensive life supports while plans were made for him to serve as an organ donor. As we thought about what Don would have told us to do, we again arrived at a clear consensus that he would want his organs donated. Keeping Don's life supports going while his organs were tested and recipients were found would be a small price to pay for this opportunity. The extra time we spent at Don's bedside was important for us as a family, since of course we were still trying to come to grips with the events that were unfolding. Once the preparations for donating Don's organs were complete, our obligation was to let him go, as hard as that was for all of us. We at least had the solace of knowing many people would now live as a result of Don's gift of organs.

This was by far the most intense end-of-life experience I have ever had. The view from the other side of the looking glass has reinforced my belief that these decisions belong as much as possible to patients and their families. As patients and families, we need medical guides who will help us fight for life when appropriate, but who also give us the information we need when that fight becomes too daunting or unwinnable. If we have to make a transition to an approach that emphasizes patient comfort, we need the commitment of these medical personnel to work with us throughout the final stages of illness all the way to death. In addition to being medical guides and partners, health care providers must also be expert listeners who can learn about the patient's personal experience and values and fully integrate them into treatment decisions. But when it comes down to hard decisions about life and death, or about which methods are acceptable or unacceptable, it is the patient's views that count the most, followed by those of the immediate family. As much as possible, the last chapter of a patient's life should be written with an eye toward the patient's own values and the circumstances of the patient's life.

In part because of the medical decisions that we made on Don's behalf, his organs will live on in the bodies of others. By reinvigorating our sense of family, Don's death will also keep us more connected to one another than would otherwise have been the case, and committed to keeping his spirit and memory alive and well for his son Dave. This is not an ending any of us would have chosen for Don, but it is the best possible outcome in the worst possible circumstances.

Index

Abortion rights, 206–207
Acceptance of bad news, 92
Acquired immunodeficiency syndrome
    (AIDS)
  delivering bad news, 78–81
  spiritual crisis, 136
  suicide risk, 89
  terminal sedation, 180–181
Active/passive distinction, 189–190
Adenocarcinoma, 215–218
Advance directives
  See also Health care proxy; Living will
Affective responses to bad news, 92–93
African-American patients
  hospice care, 72
  trust of Caucasian physicians, 20
Afterlife
  in doctor-patient relationship, 48
  near-death experiences, 11–15
  palliative care discussions, 111
Aging of population, and nonabandonment,
    60
Alaska, PAS legality, 206
"Allowing to die"
  nonabandonment, 64, 68
  U.S. vs. Dutch systems, 217–218

voluntary stopping of eating and drinking,
    179
Aloneness, 95, 111
Alzheimer's disease
  nonqualification for hospice care, 157
  palliative care for dementia, 119–131
American College of Physicians–American
    Society of Internal Medicine
  safeguards of last resort practices, 195
American Medical Association (AMA)
  Council on Ethical and Judicial Affairs,
    nonabandonment, 64
  physician-assisted suicide, 161
Amyotrophic lateral sclerosis, and
    physician-assisted suicide in Oregon,
    211
Anger, and bad news, 92, 136
Anxiety, and bad news, 92, 96
Autonomy
  delivering bad news, 86
  loss of, and physician-assisted suicide in
    Oregon, 211
  nonabandonment, 67
  palliative care discussions, 112, 206
  rule of double effect, 172
  voluntariness, 190–191

241